AF884285

THE ORIGINAL MEDICINE

A Conceptual Synopsis of Persian Medicine

Based on the Avicenna's Canon

HAMID NAMAVAR (MD., PhD)
Assistant Prof. of Traditional Medicine
Shahroud University of Medical Sciences

Shahroud University of Medical Sciences

بسم الله الرحمن الرحیم

2020 © Hamid Namavar
All Rights Reserved for the Author
All rights reserved. No part of this book may be reprinted or reproduced utilized in any form or by any electronic, mechanical, or other means now known or hereafter invented, including photocopying and recording, or in any information storage or retrieval system, without permission in writing from the author.

Title: THE ORIGINAL MEDICINE

Subtitle A Conceptual Synopsis of Persian Medicine based on the Avicenna's Canon

Author: Dr. Hamid Namavar (MD., PhD)

Cover Design: Ali Khiabanian

Publisher: American Academic Research

ISBN: 978-1947464124

The cover design of this book is the gilding of the first lithographic copy of the Avicenna's Canon of the Medicine.

CONTIBUTERS:

Mitra Mehrabani
Professor of Pharmacognosy
School of Pharmacy
Herbal and Traditional Medicines Research Center
Kerman University of Medical Sciences

Haleh Tajadini
Assistant Professor of Traditional Medicine
School of Traditional Medicine
Kerman University of Medical Sciences

Contents

PREFACE

The Persian doctrine of Medicine is a humoral medical system that deals with the management of health and diseases. It provides preventive, curative and rehabilitative healthcare with holistic approach. The fundamental framework of this system is based on deep philosophical insights and scientific principles, including the theory of four Elements; four proximate Qualities, and the theory of four Humors .Admixture of different Elements and their Qualities in specific ratio in a particular entity, whether living or non-living, denominates its Temperament. Human Temperament is commonly denoted by the dominant Humor, which can be correlated with the Temperament of Diet, Drugs, and Environmental Factors etc. as the entities of non-human Universe being made up directly of Elements are described in terms of Qualitative Temperament. Any disturbance in the equilibrium of Humors causes disease, and therefore the treatment aims at restoring the equilibrium by giving factors (including drugs) of opposite temperament. In addition, Persian doctrine of Medicine believes that *Medicatrix naturae* is the supreme power, which controls all the physiological functions of the body, provides resistance against the diseases and helps in healing naturally.

It is heartening to note that World Health Organization (WHO) since the Declaration of Alma Ata (1978) has been taking great interest in the revival of traditional Medicine including Humoral Medicine. The idea behind this was to make essential healthcare within the reach of larger sections of population worldwide at an affordable cost.

This research is a conception based on Avicenna's Cannon of medicine and has been presented as my dotoral thesis in traditional medicine; Persian medicine.

Hamid Namavar, MD., PhD.

Theories and Philosophies of Persian Medicine

Persian Medicineis based upon the theory of humors, which presupposes the presence of four humors in the body, namely blood, phlegm, yellow bile and black bile. The temperaments of persons are expressed accordingly by the words sanguine, phlegmatic, choleric and melancholic according to preponderance of the respective humor. The humors themselves are assigned temperaments. Blood is hot and moist; phlegm, cold and moist; yellow bile, hot and dry; black bile, cold and dry. Likewise, the drugs are also considered to have temperaments which are classified on the basis of their potency into grades or degrees.

In Persian Medicine, the human body is considered to comprise of the following seven components, each having a close relation with the state of health of an individual:

Arkan: States of matter and the materials entering into and forming a part of everything in the universe

Mezaj: Bodily temperament

Akhlat: Body fluids

Ruh: The vital force or life force

Qowa: The bodily powers or faculties

AF 'al: The corporeal functions

Besides, there is a residual power of self-preservation or adjustment endowed by the nature, called medicatrix naturae, which strives to restore any disturbance within the limits of the constitutional state of an individual.

States of the Body

According to Humoral physicians, states of the body are categorized in three groups as under:

(Health): in which the entire bodily functions are performed normally.

(Disease): is opposite of the health in which one or more functions or forms of the body organs are at fault.

(Neither health nor disease): the term is applied for a state of neither complete health nor disease e.g. old people or those convalescing.

Diagnostic Methods

From the very beginning, Humoral physicians have laid great emphasis on the investigation of the cause of disease and employed following means to determine the cause and nature of disease for correct diagnosis.

Pulse

Evaluation of: Quantity, Force, Duration of movement, Condition, Volume, Duration of rest period, Palpation of the pulse, Equality and inequality, Balance of the pulse, Rhythm

Physical Examination of Urine

Evaluation of: Color, Consistency, Clearness and Turbidity, Odor, Froth, Precipitates, Quantity

Physical Examination of Stool

Evaluation of: Quantity, Color, Odor, Consistency, Froth

Types of Treatment

Based on the cause and nature of disease, Persian Medicine deals with the problem through various therapeutic regimens e.g., *Regimenal Therapy, Dieto-therapy, Pharmacotherapy, manipulative techniques.*

Other Modes of Diagnosis

In addition to the above, other conventional modes of diagnosis such as Inspection, Palpation, Percussion and Auscultation have also been used by the Humoral physicians. Besides, modern tools and techniques of diagnosis are also used by Humoral physicians these days, e.g. X-ray, Ultrasound, ECG, MRI and Pathological investigations.

Prophylaxis or Prevention of Disease

Critics of Persian Medicine often claim that it does not offer anything by way of prophylaxis but the fact remains that it gives as much importance to prevention as to cure. It recognizes the influence of environment and surrounding on health and lays great emphasis on the maintenance of proper eco balance as well as pure water, food and air. Besides, it prescribes six essentials principles for maintaining good health.

Hawa' (Air)

Ma'kul-o-Mashrub (Foods and Drinks)

Harakat-o-Sukun Badani (Bodily movement and Repose)

Harakat-o-Sukun Nafsani (Psychic movement and Repose)

Nawm-o-Yaghze (Sleep and Wakefulness)

Estefragh wa Ihtebas (Evacuation and Retention)

A good Humoral physician is supposed to consider all factors before reaching a diagnosis.

Historical Background

Persian Medicine is a doctrine of healing and health maintenance in the word. The origins of Persian Medicine are found in the doctrines of the ancient Iranian physicians Rhazes and Avicenna. As a field, it was later developed and refined through systematic experiment. The history of Persian Medicine can be characterized by the work of its practitioners, or hakims, which relied on natural healing based on principles of harmony and balance, uniting the physical, mental, and spiritual realms. According to practitioners of Persian Medicine, the health of the human body is maintained by the harmonious arrangement of the seven basic physiological principles of the Persian Medicine doctrine. These principles include 1. Elements, 2. Temperament, 3. Bodily humors, 4. Organs and systems, 5. Vital spirit, 6. Faculties or powers, and 7. Functions. Interacting with each other, these seven natural components maintain the balance in the natural constitution of the human body. Each individual's constitution has a self-regulating capacity or power, called *tabiyat* (medicatrix naturae), or to keep the seven components in equilibrium.

Preface and Philosophy of Persian Medicine

Persian Medicine is a total system of healthcare, based on the original principles of medicine which were applied by Hippocrates, Galen and Ibn Sina (Avicenna), the founders of present day medicine. It includes the basic principles of modern clinical science, embracing both its theory and practice.

Persian Medicine recognises the physical, mental, emotional, and spiritual origins of both health and illness. It promotes the early diagnosis of possible pre-dispositions to diseases, well before physical symptoms appear. This prevents these diseases from appearing in a more severe form. Thereafter, treatment is integrative – combining various therapies in response to our specific needs.

Persian Medicine embraces a whole new way of looking at our body. It considers our health to be the result of a natural, harmonious balance. Persian Medicine believes that our bodies have a way of finding the path back to health. Healing comes from within. Recognition of this inherent wisdom to self-healing is essential in the treatment of disease and maintenance of health.

In this section on the Philosophy of Persian Medicine, I will cover the basic philosophical aspects of Persian Medicine, especially the main axioms of physis, temperaments, qualities, humors, and the lifestyle or governing factors. The inter-relationship between the individual and the environment, both internal and external will also be dealt with.

Definitions and Descriptions

The meaning of traditional medicine

Generally, the term *traditional medicine* refers to the art and science of preserving health, preventing illnesses and curing or alleviating disease. In traditional medicine is defined more extensively – as the science by which we learn. It embraces knowledge and understanding of:

(a) The various states of the human body, in both health and disease

(b) The means by which health is likely to be lost

(c) When lost, how health can to be restored.

This is highlighted in Ibn Sina's definition of medicine:

"Medicine is a branch of knowledge that deals with the states of health and disease in the human body for the purposes of adopting suitable measures for the preservation or restoration of health. [Ibn Sina]

Complementary medicine

There is a wide variety of medical or healing systems which are different in theory and practice to conventional medicine. These are conveniently termed complementary or alternative (to conventional medicine). The term complementary medicine is a vague and confused one in many minds. It is a general term used interchangeably with: *alternative; holistic; natural;* and *fringe*.

Many forms of complementary medicine appear, at first glance, to be completely unconnected. However, most of them are united in one important core aspect – when treating the patient, they act primarily to support the body's inner healing systems, rather than merely suppress the patient's symptoms.

Complementary medicine encourages self-healing and the prevention of disease, rather than reacting to and suppressing symptoms as they arise. In contrast, conventional medicine believes that only medicine and surgery can cure a disorder. Furthermore, conventional medicine is best at treating acute disorders, but complementary medicine has much to offer those who suffer from chronic complaints.

Common terms employed in the healthcare field

Conventional medicine: the standard scientific/medical model (or *paradigm*); also termed orthodox or allopathic medicine.

Alternative: a general term for any therapy which is used instead of conventional medicine. It can refer to systems, like Ayurveda, or to specific techniques like aromatherapy and Indian head massage.

Complementary: therapies which can be used alongside conventional medicine in order to improve the treatment outcome.

CAM: the common abbreviation for complementary and alternative medicine.

Integrative: the deliberate combination of complementary and conventional therapy in a systematic and thoughtful manner aimed at uncovering and rectifying the patient's clinical disorder.

***Holistic*:** the state of well-being in which the person's body, mind, emotions and spirit are in tune with the physical, mental, spiritual and social environment. Holistic therapy refers to treatment in which the physical, mental and social factors are taken into account, rather than just the overt diagnosed disease

***Traditional Medicine*:** is an indigenous medical belief typical of a particular region. This is often termed 'folk medicine' or 'ethno-medicine'.

Complementary medicine actually describes four separate aspects of healthcare:

- Diagnostic techniques – iridology, hair analysis, for example

- Self-help techniques – Yoga, detoxification and dieting, for example

- Therapeutic techniques – aromatherapy, hypnotherapy, for example

- Healthcare systems – Persian Medicine, Ayurveda, homeopathy, for example

Health and disease

Attaining good health is one of the biggest preoccupations of modern times. We live in a time where there is an unrelenting interest in and awareness of health-related issues. Advice on changes to our diet, the use of supplements, exotic herbs, taking more exercise, stress relieving measures and much more assail us continually, especially by the print and electronic media. Health itself, however, is not an easy concept to define.

Health is generally described in terms of either how we feel, or how capable we are of functioning. It does not merely mean not being sick, and is more than the absence of illness or unwanted physical symptoms. A person would be considered healthy if he is able to carry out his general physical, mental, occupational and social functions to his complete satisfaction. In line with this is the World Health Organisation definition:

A state of complete physical, mental and social well-being, and not merely the absence of disease or infirmity. [WHO]

However, 'healthy' usually denotes the absence of disease. According to the dictionary health is:

Freedom from bodily or mental disease or decay; a state of bodily or organic soundness; the absence of disease. [Dorland's English Dictionary]

In the Persian Medicine context health is seen as a balance between the humors which is optimal for the particular person. Health is therefore:

A state of physical, emotional, and spiritual harmony resulting from the most favourable balance of humors in a person.

Persian Medicine also believes that good health is more than the absence of symptoms. Even without troublesome symptoms, a person's ability to resist illness may be low, and his or her essential vitality may be seriously depressed.

Conventional medicine defines disease as: *A disorder with a specific cause and recognisable signs and symptoms; any bodily abnormality or failure to function properly, except that resulting directly from physical injury.* [Oxford Medical Dictionary]

This definition reveals that:

(a) Conventional medicine reduces the human body to a series of mechanistic causes and effects. A consequence of this is that patients are regarded as collections of body parts and systems, not as whole persons.

(b) Conventional medicine is primarily concerned with the physical dimension of the person. This contrasts with complementary systems, such as Persian Medicine, which place no barriers between physical, mental and spiritual well-being.

(c) Conventional medicine looks for single causes for single diseases. Complementary medicine, especially Persian Medicine, regards most if not all diseases as arising from multiple causes ('multifactorial'). These include toxins, imprudent lifestyle factors and faulty diet.

In Persian Medicine, health is present when the body's functions maintain a correct and sound balance of temperaments, structure and functions. A disease is contrary to the above – it is an abnormal condition which produces a functional disorder as a primary consequence. It can be an expression of a temperamental imbalance, humoral imbalance or a disorder of tissue structure.

Overview on Persian Medicine

Persian Medicine from the historical perspective

Avicenna believed that health is the expression of a harmonious balance between the various components of our nature, the environment that surrounds us, and our adopted lifestyle. He also believed that there is a natural and powerful tendency towards self-healing, which is driven by *Physis*. This is the body's innate vital life force, which helps to maintain the body's equilibrium or harmony, so allowing the proper functioning of the cells, tissues and organs.

During the Dark Ages in Europe, which lasted for more than 800 years, little of note was produced in the medical sphere. However, *Ibn Sina* (known in the West as *Avicenna* – "*the Prince of Physicians*") came to the fore in 980 CE. He is justifiably the most famous physician in history. Born and Resident in Persia, he was famous as a polymath, being responsible for 270 books. He codified medicine into a science in the late 10th and early 11th centuries. Persian Medicine was guarded and nurtured by Ibn Sina. He authored two major books: *The Book of Healing* and *The Canon of Medicine* – the latter being "*the single most famous book in the history of medicine*", according to the Encyclopaedia Britannica.

The Persian Medicine

For Ibn Sina, the evaluation of a disease was incomplete until all components of a person's life had been included in the diagnosis. Ibn Sina's philosophy of medicine was adopted by medieval schools of thought, and his influence on the development of medicine cannot be overstated. It has maintained its authority well over 1000 years. His *Canon of Medicine* is the textbook for Persian Medicine practitioners.

Muslim practitioners of Persian Medicine introduced, amongst others, medical botany and chemistry; organisation of the pharmacy; and the founding of hospitals, with lecture halls, charity wards, kitchens, dispensaries, qualified medical and nursing staff. Innovative techniques also appeared at this time – distillation, filtration, sublimation and calcination.

By early 1700's, the Persian Medicine system was the basis of virtually all medicine in the civilised world. It formed the basis of *Homeopathy* (developed by S. Hahnemann, 1755-1843). In the mid-1800s, Persian Medicine principles formed the basis of natural therapeutics, and these were introduced into Western medical practice.

However, the advent of homeopathy in the late 1700s, the germ theory of disease at the end of the 19th century, and the arrival of chemical or pharmaceutical medicine in the 20th century heralded major changes in medical practice.

At the present time, Persian Medicine is practiced in its original form predominantly on the Iran and Indian subcontinent. However, healing traditions directly inspired by Persian Medicine remain the treatment of choice for *around 25% of the world's present population* – over 2,000,000,000 people!

A comparison of Persian Medicine with conventional medicine is provided in the following table

	Persian Medicine	Conventional Medicine
Origin	Middle East	Europe, USA
Concepts	Physis Humors Temperament	Receptors Immune system
Elements	Earth, water, air, fire	Basic elements of nature
Cause of disease	Humoral, temperament imbalance Disturbed physis Lifestyle factors	Microbial infection Malfunctions in receptors
Diagnosis	Temperament Pulse, urine Conventional techniques, differential	Symptoms, history, physical exam, lab tests, differential, organ-related disease
Patient involvement	Empowered to make changes to diet and lifestyle	Not encouraged, not significant
Therapy objective	Support physis, restore internal balance	Suppress symptoms, kill microbes
Therapy modalities	Diet, lifestyle, herbalism, purgation, regimental therapy, etc	Antimicrobials, synthetic chemotherapy, psychotropics
Patient tolerance	Rare: side effects, overdose of herbal products	Extensive: side effects, drug interaction, overdose

Features of Persian Medicine

Background

One of the most significant features of Persian Medicine is that it is a comprehensive system of healthcare which has a sound philosophical base. This provides valuable insights into the nature of energy and matter, the origin of mankind, and the relationship that exists between humans and their environment.

Persian Medicine fully appreciates the complex interplay of our human nature, how we are all built up, and how we relate to the environment. By regarding our human nature in the broader context of the universe in which we live, we can better understand the causes of illnesses and equally important, how we can maintain optimum health.

According to Persian Medicine, a healthy person can become even healthier. It places equal emphasis on understanding the states of health and disease in the human body. Its mission is both restoring health by treating the illness, and then actively supporting the individual in maintaining optimum health.

Persian Medicine is a holistic system of healthcare

Holistic health has been defined as: "… *not merely the absence of disease or infirmity, but a state of complete physical, mental and social well-being*" [WHO].

A similar definition of holistic health has been put forward: "*the state of well-being in which an individual's body, mind, emotions and spirit are in tune with the natural, cosmic and social environment*".

Holistic medicine therefore takes into account the physical, mental, and social factors in the patient's illness, rather than just the disease that has been diagnosed. In other words, Persian Medicine has as its basic focus of activity the optimum health of the individual – not simply the absence of illness.

Another aspect of Persian Medicine and holism is that both the causes of the disorder and the susceptibility of the person to the disorder have to be addressed. For instance, in treating a person with the common cold, Persian Medicine directs its efforts into two areas; firstly, the alleviation of the symptoms (coughing, sneezing, runny nose, etc.); and secondly, enhancing the person's resistance, so that he or she is less likely to succumb to further attacks of the illness.

Persian Medicine is empirical in nature

Persian Medicine treatment is largely based on centuries of practical experience, observation and investigation. In this respect Persian Medicine differs from conventional medicine, which is more evidence-based, and is derived from experimentation according to the scientific method. For example, the use of a drug, such as a diuretic, to treat hypertension in conventional medicine follows from a number of controlled randomised clinical trials. This is the gold standard of conventional medicine. Persian Medicine, on the other hand, treats hypertension with a combination of changes to the person's lifestyle, plus the use of one or more herbal medications which have been shown effective over many years of clinical practice.

Persian Medicine does, however, accept the need for scientific enquiry. It is not only in complete harmony with the need for the basic medical sciences of biochemistry, anatomy and physiology (although interpreted in different terms such as humors, organs and members, faculties, functions and energies) but also includes the fundamentals of chemistry, physics and metaphysics.

Persian Medicine assists the natural healing process

Persian Medicine accepts that symptoms such as diarrhea, vomiting and fevers are invariably reactive responses of the body towards healing. They are often the body's attempt to rid the body of toxins which have disturbed the internal harmony. The process is directed and controlled by Physis, so is termed a *physis response*.

Persian Medicine considers that these symptoms should not be stopped, unless they have gone too far and are causing intolerable distress to the person. In other words, Physis should be supported, not suppressed. If these symptoms are actively subdued by the use of anti-diarrheal, anti-emetic and antipyretic drugs, the patient will no doubt gain relief. However, as the toxin affecting him or her has not been totally flushed from the body, the symptoms will inevitably reappear.

Persian Medicine recognises the uniqueness of the person in diagnosis and therapy

A primary feature of Persian Medicine is the concept of temperament, and its importance as part of the total diagnosis procedure. As such, Persian Medicine attaches considerable value to assessing a patient's authentic temperament as a precursor to a therapeutic approach based on his or her uniqueness, and how to restore health by supporting inner healing. In this, Persian Medicine contrasts markedly with conventional medicine, which focuses almost exclusively on diagnosing, describing and quantifying features of the patient's disorder, with scant attention paid to the individual nature of the patient. Conventional medicine treats the disease; Persian Medicine treats the person with the disease.

Persian Medicine is cost effective

Persian Medicine is ideally suited to meet the challenges of the high cost of health care. Because of the comprehensive understanding it has of the causes of illnesses, it allows for inexpensive, low-tech, easily accessible means to achieve health rather than expensive high-tech interventions. The understanding of the causes as well as the progress of diseases allows the practitioner early diagnosis of "syndromes" long before the appearance of symptoms preventing more serious diseases.

Furthermore, by advising on meaningful changes to the patient's lifestyle factors, Persian Medicine helps to reduce the chance of the disease reappearing. For example, the symptoms of type II diabetes can be readily suppressed by one or more of a number of hypoglycaemic drugs. However, this means continuous treatment, which is costly, inconvenient, and prone to side effects and probably needs regular dosage adjustment. Persian Medicine, on the other hand, will not only treat the elevated blood sugar, but will counsel on lifestyle changes which will result in the underlying conditions that lead to the illness in the first place being resolved.

Persian Medicine supports integrative medicine as a route to optimum health

Integrative (or integrated) medicine is:

"The deliberate practice of medicine that selectively incorporates concepts, values and practices of complementary, alternative and conventional medicine into comprehensive diagnosis and treatment plans."

It is not just a mixture of conventional medicine and another healthcare system such as Persian Medicine. Rather, it emphasises wellness and healing of the entire person as the primary outcomes, rather than disease and therapy. It regards the patient in his or her entirety, not only as a physical body, but with mental and spiritual dimensions as well. All of these are recognised, and involved in diagnosis and treatment whenever appropriate.

Furthermore, integrative medicine is concerned with encouraging individual responsibility for one's own health, and tries to avoid the more authoritarian approach generally adopted in conventional medicine. Integrative medicine, therefore, is a partnership of equals, with the patient and the practitioner involved in the development and implementation of a comprehensive treatment plan, not just resolving the patient's immediate disorder.

Conventional medicine tends to look for a single cause (such as microbes, toxins or biochemical abnormalities) as being responsible for a particular disorder. In contrast, an important feature of integrative medicine is that it considers that disease arises from a number of causes (that is, 'multifactorial'), often embracing genetic, physical, emotional, psychological, and spiritual factors. The integrative medical approach therefore seeks to identify multiple origins of a disease, and, ideally, address them all as necessary. As a result, the range of options in the practice of integrative medicine can go beyond standard conventional therapeutic practice. It can become involved in the patient's spiritual life and social relationships, employ mind-body practices, and combine this with the use of herbs, physical manipulative techniques techniques and surgery.

Persian Medicine clearly accepts and defines the complex integration between the many organs and tissues of the body, and understands how organs and systems of the body influence each other. This complete integration is well understood under the three organ theory which fully explains the relationship that exists between the different parts of the body. This theory recognizes and accepts the interrelationship between different organs and systems of the body which influences the outcome of disease and needs to be taken into account when treatment is applied.

Persian Medicine empowers and involves the patient in therapy

Persian Medicine emphasises empowerment of the patient as well as preventative medicine. Here again, the understanding of the causes of diseases enables the practitioner to advise his patients more effectively on management of illnesses and primary health care.

The Macrocosm and the Microcosm

As we now know, everything in the Universe (or *Macrocosm*) is interconnected in one way or another. We as individuals do not exist in our own self-contained world (or *Microcosm*), but are connected to other parts of the Macrocosm: via our behaviour in our families, our communities, our societies, our planet, and our very existence.

The approach by conventional medicine	***The Persian Medicine approach***
1. The body is regarded as a complex machine	Persian Medicine deals with the whole patient
2. The body and mind are seen as separate entities	The body, mind and spirit are interconnected
3. Emphasises the elimination of disease	Emphasises ways of achieving good health
4. Treat the symptoms troubling the patient	Treats the underlying causes of the disorder
5. Specialises – diseases of the heart, kidney, etc.	Takes an integrated, holistic approach
6. Use high-tech, impersonal diagnostic techniques, and heroic therapeutic measures	Focuses on diet, lifestyle, and preventative measures and intuition based on experience
7. Focuses on objective information (how the patient is doing – charts, tests, statistics)	Focus on subjective information (how the patient is feeling)
8. The physician is emotionally neutral and detached	The Persian Medicine physician's care and empathy are critical to healing
9. The physician is the all-knowing, unchallengeable authority	The physician is a partner with the patient in the healing process
10.The physician is in control of the patient's health problems	The patient is in charge of health care choices
11.The physician treats disease	The Persian Medicine physician promotes health (physician is a nature server)

As human beings, we are all ulimately made up of the same basic material as the rest of the Universe. We connect with the Macrocosm by our behaviour, our actions, and even the air that we breathe. We influence all living organisms which share the earth with us.

Harmony

A harmonious balance normally exists between the components of the Macrocosm, whether at the cosmic, geological, social or physiological levels. The relationship between the fauna and flora, man and animals, the atmosphere, the oceans, and the earth are all carefully and delicately balanced for the maintenance and perpetuation of life. An example of the maintenance of this balance for the perpetuation of life on this planet is seen if we consider on the salt content in the sea. Despite the natural disasters of earthquakes, volcanic eruptions or the effect of mankind extracting salt from the sea over thousands of years, the saline content in the oceans is still ideal for all forms of marine life.

This harmonious balance is guided by an organizing principle, the *Supreme Wisdom of the Universe,* the essence of which exists in every living entity. This inherent wisdom resides in our genetic makeup (our genes), and in our folk memories (our memes). This inherent wisdom is recognised in several medical philosophies and disciplines, such as Chinese Herbal Medicine, Ayurvedic Medicine and Homeopathy. In Persian Medicine, this inherent wisdom is called *physis (medicatrix naturea).*

The Concept of Physis (Medicatrix Naturea)

Description

"Nature heals, and the physician is only nature's assistant"

Our health can be regarded as an expression of a dynamic but harmonious balance between the various components of our nature, our environment, and our lifestyle. Physis is the intrinsic ability of the body to preserve health, and the mechanism that activates the body's healing processes.

Briefly stated, physis is the vital life force, inherent in the human body, which helps to maintain equilibrium or harmony within the internal environment, so allowing the proper functioning of the cells, tissues and organs. In addition, it regulates the reservoir of energy which is the driving force behind maintaining homeostasis in the myriad of complex processes we recognise as life. It is the origin of movement and rest.

The various systems in the body – the circulatory, respiratory, digestive, immune systems, etc. – have their own organisation. However, they do not work in complete isolation, but are each connected to the other systems in order to function effectively and efficiently. In the human being, physis has the innate ability to orchestrate the body into maintaining dynamic optimum functioning, better known as *homeostasis*. It acts to heal the body when it is sick, restore it when it is depleted, and to develop and thrive when supplied with suitable nourishment. As the regulator for homeostasis, it is essentially the human's 'inborn intelligence of health'.

In the event of disease (or even when the body fails to reach its ideal state), physis acts to correct imbalances and disharmony. One important feature of physis is that it operates in all dimensions of health – in the physical, the emotional, the spiritual, and, arguably, the social.

Physis and other medical philosophies

Physis is recognised in other healing philosophies – as *Prana* (Ayurvedic Medicine); *Chi Energy* (Chinese Medicine); the *Vital Force* (Complementary Medicine); the *Life Force* (Homeopathic Medicine), and *Nature* (Naturopathy). Hippocrates described it as *Medicatrix Naturae*. Physis is also akin to the *Yin and Yang* principle of oriental philosophy. It has also been termed the *Divine Wisdom* and even *Mother Nature*.

In early Western holistic medicine, it was labelled the *Etheric Body*. It has also been variously described as the *Vital Force, naturae* and the *Hierarchical Principle.* Physis was used to describe the natural vitality of what is now recognised as the immune system, in its spontaneous response to environmental influences. It was quickly brought into action to detect and react to both supportive and disruptive factors. In fact, one component of physis is our immunological identity, which forms the molecular basis of healing. Another aspect of physis, which is a key focus of the relatively new discipline of psycho-neuro-immunology (PNI), is the placebo response, and the possibly associated phenomenon of spontaneous healing.

"When physis is powerful enough to withstand the disease, it does not require the aid of the physician, as in the case of minor diseases that are self-healing" [Al-Malki]

The nature of physis

Physis comes into effect from the instant of fertilisation, and is present until the moment of death. It maintains harmony between the individual and both the internal and the external environments. Physis ensures that an ideal balance exists within the body's cells, in the tissues, between the many internal organs, and the entire body. This dynamic maintenance of harmony within the body is also termed *homeostasis,* mentioned earlier.

Physis is the administrator of the body, and it operates for in the physical, mental and spiritual dimensions.

In the *physical context*, physis ensures that the many millions of biochemical reactions taking place – for protection, for growth, tissue maintenance, reproduction and repair – which are taking place at any instant, are controlled. Physis embraces all metabolic and homeostatic functions of the body.

At the *psychological level*, the harmony or balance of the complex of emotions, the control of destructive urges or thoughts, and the maintenance of good mental health is regulated by Physis.

One specific aspect of physis relevant in health and disease is *the immune system*. This ensures that infections arising from outside do not disturb the body's internal harmony. It also maintains an extensive surveillance on the body's many tissues, to detect any cancers in development, and remove them if they become established.

Other aspects of Physis in the physiological dimension are the numerous *biochemical feedback* mechanisms which operate in the body's metabolic processes, and *the endocrine regulation* of hormone secretion from glands.

Physis is not confined to humans – it pervades all living tissue: it is part of the *biochemical unity of life*. It follows the laws of nature as we understand them, and works in a pre-determined, instinctual manner.

Physis and medicine

The word *"physician"* is derived originally from the word *physis*. The true role of the physician is to aid physis in the healing process, by understanding the factors governing physis, and plan and execute treatment accordingly. For example, when a person has eaten something that disagrees with him or her, then vomiting or diarrhea is a natural reaction. The physician should be aware of this natural reaction, and assist physis by devising effective treatment which is in harmony with the body's healing mechanisms. Treatment comes from outside; healing from within.

Behind every natural action of the human body is an inherent wisdom, a mechanism [physis] that allows the body to heal itself. In fact, no herb, no food or any other substance or procedure can do anything on its own to heal. It can only assist the body in its own self-healing role. If your finger is cut, it is not the stitches or the bandage or the iodine that causes it to heal; it is the skin itself that performs this miracle.

There are two situations which physis corrects changes in a person's temperament:

1. Changes in a person's qualities. This may arise from changes in the environment, personal behaviour, diet and other lifestyle factors.

2. Changes to actual changes in matter. This involves qualitative or quantitative changes to humoral composition.

Temperament, structure and function

According to Persian Medicine philosophy, every part of the human being has been created with a specific shape and structure in order to fulfil a specific function.

For example:

- The shape of ears enhances our ability to hear.

- Our nose filters out impurities from inspired air before it enters the lungs.

- Our eyebrows prevent perspiration from entering our eyes.

When examining the geometry of our internal organs, we see many different shapes, again performing different functions, each having a specific temperament. For example, the shape of the heart facilitates the pumping action whereas the overall temperament of the brain is moist (with less heat), enabling nerve impulses to be transmitted easily, because moisture is a good conductor of electrical impulses. On the other hand, the overall temperament of the liver is hot (with less moistness), because of the heat generated during the process of metabolism.

Delving further into the marvels of the body, we begin to realise just how intricate the systems of the body are: the respiratory, the circulatory, and the digestive systems, and of special significance in the context of health and disease, the Immune system. Each system working independently and yet is associated with and interconnected to each other.

The human body is unbelievably complex. It has been created with self-regulatory, self-healing mechanisms that are under the control of physis. This governing principle maintains the correct structure and temperament of the body and its components, in order to perform the desired functions. Every cell, tissue and organ is in equilibrium with its characteristic primary qualities, or temperament, upon which its structure and functions depends.

Changes in both structure and temperament will affect functions. These changes can occur from the qualitative effects of the interaction of man and his environment. As we are part of the universe, things that happen outside our bodies have an influence on us. As everything in the universe possesses qualities, whether in the form of energy or matter, qualities are the common link within the universe.

Qualities

As everything in the universe is made up of primary matter with corresponding qualities, the effect that qualities have on human beings as well as all living organisms is an important consideration in Persian Medicine. Whether we are conscious of them or not, we are constantly experiencing them and being influenced by them.

According to the dictionary,

Quality is a distinctive attribute or property which gives individuality.

In Persian Medicine, the qualities comprise of Heat, Coldness, Dryness and Moistness:

The qualities *Heat* and *Moistness* are said to be the *active qualities.*

The qualities *Coldness* and *Dryness* are said to be the *passive qualities.*

To understand the influence that these qualities have on us it is necessary to understand the interaction of qualities in nature.

The quality of *heat* will have an effect opposite that of *coldness*; and the quality of *moistness* will have an effect opposite that of *dryness*.

Opposing qualities cannot exist simultaneously. Nothing can be hot and cold at the same time, nor moist and dry at the same time.

Combination of qualities

The qualities of heat, coldness, moistness and dryness interact with each other in Nature; in such a way that one active quality and one passive quality combine to give rise to a compound qualitative effect. For example, *Hot and Moist*, or *Cold and Moist*, or *Cold and Dry*, or *Hot and Dry*

Temperament and Healthcare

Background

Each one of us is unique. But what is the essence of this uniqueness? The basis of the human temperament, and why it fluctuates so much between people of similar background and upbringing, and even between people in the same family, has been a source of fascination for thousands of years. Every age has a preferred explanation of the obvious differences amongst people, and many have attributed the differences to physiology – in ancient times to bodily fluids, and more recently, to genes. The subject of a person's individuality or uniqueness – what is called *temperament* in Persian Medicine – is now going through a revival of interest, for three good reasons:

(a) Because of what we now know about our behaviour during personal development;

(b) Because of our varying responses to medical intervention; and

(c) Because the technological advancements with the computer age have enabled better understanding of the bio-chemistry and genetics of the human body.

Persian Medicine and temperament

The diagnosis of a person's temperament is a major pre-requisite for accurate diagnosis and effective therapy when practicing Persian Medicine. This has been highlighted when he mentioned:

"*It is more important to know what sort of a person has a disease than to know what sort of disease a person has*"

Temperament is a term which describes a person's physical characteristics (the *constitution*) plus his or her psychological, emotional, and spiritual attributes. It assesses personality strengths and weaknesses, and includes the predisposition (*risk factors*) for particular disorders.

Persian Medicine therefore attaches considerable importance to assessing a patient's authentic temperament, as it is an important precursor to a therapeutic approach based on his or her uniqueness, and how to restore health by supporting inner healing. In this, Persian Medicine contrasts markedly with the conventional medical system, which focuses almost exclusively on diagnosing, describing and quantifying features of the patient's presenting disorder, with little attention paid to the patient's uniqueness or individuality.

The human body is an unbelievably complex biological system, probably beyond our capacity to understand fully. It is based on a vast array of self-regulatory and self-healing mechanisms, operating at the cellular, tissue and organ level, which are under the control of Physis. This maintains the correct structure and temperament for the person, so allowing him or her to perform the functions necessary to maintain health and prevent disease.

Changes in structure or temperament will affect the body's functions. These may occur as a result of an interaction with the environment.

The practice of Persian Medicine revolves around the art and skill of identifying a person's individual authentic temperament, combined with the science and practice of serving his or her Physis to reach and maintain their particular ideal state of health.

Temperamental Types

Although the number of possible temperaments is virtually infinite, Persian Medicine has narrowed them down to the four temperamental types: sanguineous, phlegmatic, melancholic and choleric.

As well as different people being divided into the four temperamental types above, each temperamental type also has a combination of qualities associated with it.

Therefore, each temperamental type also has different qualities assigned to them:

Sanguineous – the qualities of hot and moist

Phlegmatic – the qualities of cold and moist

Choleric– the qualities of hot and dry

Melancholic – the qualities of cold and dry

Humors

An important concept in Persian Medicine is the humoral theory. The humors are the primary fluids that are manufactured from the digestion of food and drink, which are processed and transformed in the liver. Every level of organisation within the body is infused by and interconnected with the humors. A proper balance of humors ensures efficient metabolism, and prevents the build-up of toxins. Humors give rise to all constituents of the body. Also, a person's temperament is maintained by the balance of humors within. They are the agents which form the bridge linking the microcosm of the human body to the macrocosm of the universe.

Humors are very much involved in the origin and development of a particular illness, the diagnostic principles invoked, and the therapeutic approaches adopted in the healing process.

Historically, the core concept of humors was originated by Hippocrates, expanded by Galen, and formalised by Ibn Sina and his medical contemporaries, who completed the final classification, codification and application of Persian Medicine. The theory of humors fits comfortably into the physics of primary matter or four elements (air, water, earth, and fire) and four qualities (hot, cold, dry, and moist).

There are four humors, with different qualities:

• Blood – sanguineous humor [*dam*] (Qualities: *Hot and Moist*)

• Phlegm – phlegmatic humor [*balgham*] (Qualities: *Cold and Moist*)

• Yellow bile – bilious humor [*safra*] (Qualities: *Hot and Dry*)

• Black bile – melancholic humor) [*sauda*] (Qualities: *Cold and Dry)*

The humors can also be regarded from a more metaphysical standpoint. In his translation of the "*Canon of Medicine*", O.C. Gruner states that:

"Humor should not be regarded as matter, but more as "*an essence*" or "*quasi-material*" that make up the body fluids.

The metaphysical nature of humors is similar to and associated with the four primary matters of earth, water, air and fire. Both primary matter and humors have assigned qualities which are in essence the link between energy and matter.

For example, whilst humors are produced by the liver from food and drink, the food and drink also provides the primary matter component that translates into body fluids containing minerals, amino acids, hormones, enzymes, etc.

Gruner also states that:

"In a sense the body fluids are the meeting places of various opposing forces and/or primary matter."

Humors together with the body fluids form the basis of all cells from which tissues are formed. The humors, although metaphysical, influence the outcome of the physical manifestations of the body fluids. This includes the cells, tissues, organs and ulimately the entire human being.

The humors have three main functions:

1. Maintaining the *temperamental balance* (qualitatively).

2. Providing *nutrition* for the maintenance of the body's complex structure by replacing body's tissues.

3. Provides the *energy requirements* for the various activities of the body.

Homeostasis between temperament and humors

The human being is a dynamic entity interacting physically, (in the form of catabolism and anabolism) intellectually, emotionally and spiritually. The humors are responsible for ensuring that the ideal qualitative state or temperament of the individual is maintained according to his/her ideal requirements.

The four humors exist in an individual in different combinations. This ensures that the overall qualitative state of the humors is in harmony with the overall qualitative state of the individual. For example, if a person has a dominant sanguineous and sub-dominant phlegmatic temperament, the person's overall qualitative and quantitative ratio will have an overall quality that has more *moisture*, then *heat*, then *coldness* and then the least, *dryness*. This will be ensured by an overall comparative dominance of sanguineous humor over the others in this individual.

This ideal state can be altered both *qualitatively* (changes in qualities of heat, coldness, moistness and dryness) and *quantitatively* (changes in the ratios of the humors).

Health will only be maintained as long as the overall quality of the humors is in harmony with the overall quality of the individual's temperament. The qualities of the diet consumed and the effects of the environment constantly influence and alter the qualities in the humor.

The primary matter (elements), humors and temperaments can be summarised

The Primary matter (elements)	**AIR**	**WATER**	**EARTH**	**FIRE**
The Qualities	Hot & Moist	Cold & Moist	Cold & Dry	Hot & Dry
The Temperaments	Sanguineous	Phlegmatic	Melancholic	Bilious
The Humors	Sanguineous	Phlegmatic	Melancholic	Bilious

The functioning of the human being

This is illustrated in the diagram on the following page. In this we see that the metaphysical humors, together with the primary matters and their respective qualities, become the basis for the physical matter. This ranges from organic compounds, to sub-cellular organelles, to cells, tissues, body organs, organ complexes and ulimately the total human being. This represents the physical, emotional, intellectual and spiritual components of the human being. The humors are responsible for ensuring that at every level of organisational growth the correct temperament is achieved and maintained.

Tissues and Organs

The humors or body fluids form the building blocks for the four major types of tissues – connective tissue, muscular tissue, epithelial tissue and nervous tissue.

Different organs are made up of different ratios of these tissues.

Compound Organs

Compound organs are a combination of the different tissues; for example, heart, lungs, liver, pancreas, stomach and brain all have their own individual temperament.

The compound organs are divided into three main groups under the control of the three main organs the heart (animistic), liver (vital) and the brain (psychic).

Animistic– these are the organs of the cardiovascular and respiratory system, all of which are controlled by the heart

Vital – these are the organs associated with the digestive and excretory systems, all of which are "controlled" by the liver. The reproductive organs can also be included in this group.

Psychic – these are the organs of the central and peripheral nervous system, all of which are controlled by the brain.

Energy, Faculties and Function

Energies

According to Persian Medicine, what a thing is – its essential nature – is closely related to what it does – its function.

The power of an object to behave or function in a certain way and to produce particular effects is thought to reveal the basic nature of that object. This power is derived from the inherent wisdom within the object, and is called a *faculty*.

However, in order for the faculties to perform their functions, energy is required.

After food has been ingested, digested and metabolised, humors are formed in the liver, with the assistance of inspired oxygen. These humors then act as nutrients for the formation, development and maintenance of cells, tissues and organs.

The energy is produced by *oxidative respiration* – from the interaction between the oxygen inhaled and the subsequent conversion of glucose into adenosine tri-phosphate (ATP), also known as the 'energy currency' of living tissues. The faculties of the body will continue their functions as long as adequate energy, as ATP, remains available to the respective organs. This energy is used by the three faculties (*see below*) to carry out their specific, pre-determined functions.

Faculties and functions

There are three basic faculties within the human body:

- The animistic faculty
- The vital faculty
- The Psychic faculty

The seat of the animistic faculty is the *heart.*

- It regulates the *immune system*;
- It controls *muscle tissue.*

The animistic faculty performs its functions by the processes of breathing and the functioning of the heart.

The seat of the vital faculty is the *liver.*

• It regulates the *endocrine/exocrine system*;

• It controls the *epithelial tissue.*

The vital faculty performs its function of metabolism through its *attractive, retentive, digestive and repulsive* inherent capabilities that exist within this faculty.

The seat of the Psychic faculty is the *brain.*

• It regulates the *nervous system*;

• It controls the *nervous tissue.*

The psychic faculty performs its function through the perceptive (sensory) afferent nerves of the external senses of sight, hearing, sense, smell and touch and the internal senses of cognitive, memory, thinking, common sense and imagination.

Having discussed the constitution of the human being from the Persian Medicine perspective, that is, primary matter, temperament, humors, organs and tissues, energies, faculties and functions, we see the relationship between the Persian Medicine constitution of the human being and the basic sciences of biochemistry, anatomy and physiology as follows.

The Lifestyle Factors

Background

Hippocrates firmly believed in the interaction of living organisms, especially human beings, with the external environment. He felt that we take from the environment the nutrients and other factors which help us grow, develop and survive, and return to the environment the waste products rejected by the body.

The efficient interaction with the environment and the ability to effectively 'digest' the environment constitutes health.

According to Persian doctrine of medicine disease is as a result of the difficulty in the digestion or '*pepsis*', of the environment, by the organism. The term of *dyspepsia* is still used today.

However, the understanding of '*dyspepsia*' extended beyond the inability to digest food and drink but extended to the effective digestion of the total environment in a state of complete harmony.

Our personal health reflects the extent to which this interaction is successful; if we fail to derive adequate nutrition from our environment, then we will fail to thrive. Also, if we are inefficient in rejecting unwanted, waste products, then our very survival will be threatened by a build-up of toxic materials.

According to Persian Medicine, our health reflects a state of harmony with our personal environment. Central to the preservation of health is the correct maintenance of the innate heat, and the conservation of moisture in the body. Their harmony is affected by the normal human activities of breathing, eating and drinking, sleeping, bodily evacuation, movement and rest. The emotional state and age of the person, together with the season of the year will also exert an effect.

Any disease is ulimately a symptom of our failure to assimilate and use the various environmental factors effectively. These factors include the air we breathe, and the food and drink we consume. However, there are several other factors present in the environment (which are now being re-discovered) that are capable of influencing our health, both for better, or for worse.

Persian Medicine has identified a number of lifestyle factors (also termed '*governing factors*') which profoundly influence our health. How we respond to these factors – *how we allow them to flow through us* – determines how we grow, move, think and feel.

Management of the lifestyle factors determines the outcome of health or disease. If well managed, good health will be maintained; if poorly managed, disease will result.

The lifestyle factors in health and disease

The *six essential lifestyle factors* are:

- Environmental air and breathing
- Food and drink
- Movement and rest
- Our emotional life
- Sleep and wakefulness
- Elimination and retention

The effects of the six lifestyle factors are translated by the qualities of heat, moistness, coldness and dryness they increase or decrease.

For example, the weather can be hot, cold, moist or dry; foods have inherent qualities within them which can be either heating or cooling, and with moistness or dryness (heating foods increases metabolic rate and cooling foods decrease it). Similarly, movement increases heat, resting confers a cooling effect, and emotions (such as anger) also produce heat. Sleeping cools the person down, increasing moisture.

These external factors were originally called the "*non-naturals*", because they affected the body from the *outside*. They were said to have numerous inevitable effects on the person, for good or bad. If the person was 'intemperate' in any or several of these, then disease would certainly follow.

Ibn Sina referred to these lifestyle factors as the "governing factors", as he felt they have a governing effect on our state of health and vulnerability to disease. The terms 'lifestyle factors' and 'governing factors' are used interchangeably.

For health to be maintained, all six governing factors need to be regulated. This regulation comes under the heading of 'hygiene' in its widest sense.

The six lifestyle factors are not equally important, nor needed to the same extent, for every person. A person's temperament decides what quality and quantity of each lifestyle factor is necessary to maintain the optimum balance, and the manner this can be achieved.

In Persian Medicine, the practitioner must also personally apply the rules of good hygiene, if he or she is to assess and understand the patient correctly.

Seven Natural Principles in Persian Medicine

Humoral Theory

The theory supposes the presence of four humors in the body (blood, phlegm; yellow-bile and black-bile). Temperaments of individuals are expressed according to the preponderance of humors (these may be sanguine, phlegmatic choleric and melancholic respectively). The humors themselves are assigned temperaments. As the individuals are assigned specific temperaments, likewise animals, minerals and drugs (natural) are assigned temperaments and their orders (standards) are considered in the light of their pharmacological potential (or efficacy). This brief concept can be tabulated as under

Humors	**temperament**	**individual's temperament**
blood	Hot & moist	sanguine
phlegm	cold & moist	phlegmatic
yellow bile	Hot & dry	choleric
black bile	cold & dry	melancholic

These humors, like everything else in the world of nature, are composed of the elements and natures in different mixtures, proportions and combinations.

Including therefore humors (which constitute the building units of the body and are considered as the primary body-fluids produced from digested food) there are seven fundamental theoretical and functional principles regarding the human body:

- Elements (arkaan) comprising different stages of matter and materials entering into and forming a part of everything in the universe (Elementary constituents)

- The body temperament (mezaj) (biochemical/ physicochemical constituents)

- Humors (akhlat) - the structural components (active fluid constituents)

- The fully developed mature organs(aza) (anatomical constituents)

- The vital force, or life-force (rooh)

- The bodily power (ghova) (Potential or kinetic energy)

- Functions (afaal)(the corporeal functions, physiological processes).

Among them, the first three are the theoretical principles which have entered into the phase of determination, distinction and analysis, whereas the other four constitute the somatic orientation of body, among them 5th (rooh) is identified as pneuma or Spirit.

The major contribution of Avicenna is that he:

- established the fact that disease was a natural process

- made people realize that symptoms were the reaction of body to disease(s)

- First time introduced the idea that the chief function of physician was to activate the natural forces of the body (to act against disease).

Avicenna is credited to have transformed medicine from the mixture of empirical, pseudo-scientific and superstitious into science. He freed medicine from the surcingle of superstition on one hand and from the philosophical speculation on the other hand. The greatest contribution of Avicenna's medicine - indeed is to relate the cause to the effect and to discover the points of similarities in the classification of diseases and thereby placing diagnostic treatment on sound basis.

According to Avicenna the human body was composed of four humors - blood, phlegm, black-bile and yellow- bile, an equilibrium of which meant health, and a disequilibrium ensue disease. Avicenna stated:

"Concerning the composite parts of man's body, it has blood, phlegm, yellow-bile and black-bile. These make up his parts and through them he suffers illness or enjoys health. When all of these elements are truly balanced and mingled in proper ratios, he feels the most perfect health. Illness occurs when one of these qualities is in excess or is lowered in amount or is entirely eliminated from the body. Because when one of these elements is isolated so that it has no balance with one or the others, the particular part of the body, where it is supposed to make balance, naturally becomes diseased."

Thus matter (comprising elementary constitution) in its different states and forms helped by the temperaments (mezaj) of its individual constituents produces humors (akhlaat) or the structural components of the body. Their different components combine to produce the organs (aza); and the life-spirits (arvaah). The organs with the help of spirit or pneuma develop energy (ghova) which is made to manifest itself in the actions (afaal) of the body.

Details about each of the above categories will be discussed subsequently.

Medicatrix Naturae

According to Persian Medicine, every person is supposed to have a unique humoral constitution which represents his healthy state. Any change in this constitution brings about a change in his state of health. There is formulated also a bower of self-preservation or adjustment (Medicatrix Naturae) which strives to restore any disturbance within the limits prescribed by the constitution or state of the individual.

Great reliance is placed on this bower, the aim of the physician being able to help restore and develop rather than supersede or impede the action of this bower. The consequence of this act is that by the use of Persian Medicine not only is the system enabled to overcome the present disturbance under the force of intrinsic bower already available in the body but it also emerges, after recovery, with greater bower of resistance to future disturbances. In case of emergencies or immediate daily life sufferings of common origin, simples' (mofradat) use is advised which are usually available from the stock of house hold remedies. Persian Medicine actually helps this bower of self-preservation either by re-activating it directly or by assisting it against specific disease situations.

Expressing his opinion about the Avicenna's theory of humors, was stated:

It was a highly workable theory and explained a great deal. Each humor had elementary qualities. Thus blood was hot and moist like air, phlegm was cold and moist like water, and yellow-bile was hot and dry like earth, whereas black-bile corresponds with the availability of element identified as fire - the cosmic element. Man was part of nature. Nature was constituted by the four elements, the human body by the four humors, and elements and humors had their elementary qualities in common. They formed the bridge between the microcosm (Individual) and the macrocosm (Universe).

When the humors were normal in quality and quantity and well mixed so that the condition of eukrasia prevailed, man was healthy. However, as a result of disturbances, one humor came to dominate in an abnormal way, the balance was upset, the mixture lost equilibrium, a dyskrasia prevailed and the individual was sick. What happened was that the organism, by virtue of its innate healing power which later was called the ***Medicatrix Naturae,*** endeavored to restore the balance. The humors, which were considered crude in beginning of the disease, underwent a process of ripening, a coaction; and when they had matured, the faulty matter, was driven out in the urine, the stools, sputum or as pus. Where upon the balance was restored and the patient cured? On the other hand, if the disturbance was such that the natural process could not overcome it, the patient succumbed. The very important practical consequence of these views was that the physician was taught to direct his entire treatment in such a way that it would assist the innate healing power of the body and avoid whatever might possibly antagonize it. He did this by prescribing an appropriate diet, the effect of which could be enhanced by drugs. However, in certain cases, he took recourse to the surgical procedures. By opening an abscess, he helped nature to drive out the pus (and by venesection he assisted quick draining of blood containing mal humors which have entered into its composition and deposited, or have become the cause of any specific humor's decline in the blood composition), thus shortening the process and saving the forces of the organism.

The humors had elementary (qualities) and (since they determined the character of the diseases, these had) also dominating qualities. Drugs, too, like other objects of nature, had definite qualities, specific temperaments and thus a disease that was Hot and moist was to be cured by drugs that were cold and dry. Physicians have well-differentiated between four degrees of intensity. The theory of four humors could also be used to explain the various constitutional types of humans. No two individuals are the same, but one can distinguish certain groups. They are tall and short, fat and lean, intelligent and dumb, irascible (irritable and hot- tempered) and sullen (ill-humored, moody). It was observed in antiquity that certain physical and mental qualities occur in definite combinations. Stout persons are usually good-natured. The devil is never pictured as fat, for this would have made him a good devil! (Possibly the healthy- one). The humoral theory seemed to explain these differences. It was assumed that one of the four humors could slightly dominate physiologically without causing disease. Thus, if black-bile (normal cold & dry temperament) dominated the individual belonged to the melancholic type. It was the type to which many men of genius belonged-philosophers, statesmen, and artists; but there was a somewhat imbalanced type which today we could call maniac-depressives, the people who Somtimes are in high spirits and Somtimes deeply depressed. Similarly, it was assumed that blood, phlegm, and yellow-bile could dominate physiologically and so the physicians describe the sanguine, phlegmatic and choleric types.

The theory of four humors had a most prolonged influence on medical thought and it illustrated graphically the philosophical interpretations of disease. The humoral theory was the result of many brilliant and correct observations. It was logical, explained many phenomena of health and disease, and has valuable guidance to the medical practitioner, and it was not scientific in our sense of the word: nobody had ever seen the black-bile and the qualities Hot, cold, dry, moist were not physical concepts.

Scientific experiments were conducted in biology too, but the scientific means (as to explain or observe humors in physical sense) were not available for a physical interpretation of health and disease, and the need for a comprehension of these phenomena was satisfied by logical philosophic speculations.

An eminent exponent of Persian Medicine, Hakim Mostafavi Kashani, has this to say about the theory of temperament:

Not long ago many modem physicians ridiculed the theory of temperament (based on humors). They put it aside as an irrelevant off-shoot of ancient medicine. But now various branches of medicine, notably immunology, genetics, cytology, hematology and psychosomatic medicine etc., have begun to support the theory. These branches have unearthed the truth that as there are differences in the appearance of features of individuals, there is also a specific temperament having its own individual characteristics. Evidently, in order to deal with the problem of health of a person, some specific treatment is necessary. It appears that the day is not far- off when cards of patients will also contain notes about their temperament and laws of treatment in addition to the record of their sensitivity to antibiotics and chemotherapeutic agents. When this happens, the method of mass treatment (through chemotherapy alone) will have to be discarded.

Revival of Herbal medicine, conservation of the nature and preservation of health, keeping in view the sanctity of the environment and the individual, as well as utilizing the available natural resources (instead of ultra-specific treating agents) through alternative systems of medicine, to alleviate disease on the micro- as well as macrosomic levels, all such contributions point towards realization of the fact that Holistic Approach is the most significant of all tactics being exploited to rescue today's human being from the clutches of ailments and diseases.

Prevention of Disease

Persian Medicine aims at restoring the equilibrium of various elements and faculties of the human body. It presupposes the presence of a remedial nature in the human system and attempts to call it into action to restore the normal health. Persian Medicine has recognized the influence of surroundings and ecological conditions on the state of health of human beings. It has laid down six essentials and has put greater emphasis on the one hand, on the maintenance of proper ecological balance, and on the other hand, keeping the water, food and air free from all pollution. The essentials, known in Persian Medicineas "*six essential factors*" include:

Air, Water, Food and Drinks, Bodily movements and repose, Sleep and wakefulness, and Evacuation and retention

Therapeutics

The term “elaaj“ means the science of treatment or curative procedures.

This science is divided into three main branches: Regimental therapy, pharmacotherapy, manipulative techniques

Regimental therapy

This category of treatment covers a wide range of special techniques and physical means and processes of generally simple nature. The concept of this manner of treatment is ***capture in six essential factors***. These include, sweating, diuresis, the use of baths, exercise, purging, vomiting, dietotherapy and etc.

Diet plays a more important role in Persian Medicine than in modern medicine. Consuming the right food and drink and in the right amount as well as in the right manner is one of the six essentials of sound health. In the view of physicians, the effect of diet on both health and illness is generally more powerful than that of drugs.

The scientific basis of dietotherapy, according to Persian Medicine, is the theory of correspondence between the natures within the humors of the body and the natures in food. Like drugs and humors, food possesses various natures in different degrees, thereby affecting the humoral constitution of the person who consumes it. Accordingly, dietotherapy seeks to cure certain diseases by regulating the dietary habits of the patient. Since the fundamental idea of therapeutics in Persian Medicine is to find a medicine which can aid the body's natural power of self-preservation (Is called ***Medicatrix Naturae***) to fight-off the disease in question. The task of a physician is also to prescribe a diet that's nutritive and pharmacological properties are capable of strengthening the individual body's natural power or what we now call immune system. The following remarks by a contemporary nutritionist and naturopath are very much in the spirit of Persian Medicine: "We know that the human body has all sorts of weapons at its disposal to fight-off invading germs. There are many factors affecting functions of these weapons including previous exposure to similar germs, heredity stress, emotions and nutrition."

Pharmacotherapy

This is a field in which Persian Medicine system possesses a remarkable wealth of knowledge and made many outstanding contributions to the advancement of medicine. Here the principles of pharmacology and pharmacotherapy are related to the humoral theory of medicine. The use of a particular drug is governed by three main factors:

- The nature of the drug in question.
- The nature of the ailment in question, and
- The temperament of the patient.

The guiding principle is that the drug to be prescribed should possess qualities opposite to those present in the disease in question.

Iranian literature on pharmacology contains a detailed view of the following:

- The nature, qualities, and temperament of drugs
- Gradation of the potency of drugs (orders)
- Division of drugs according to quality (pharmacological classification)
- Action of drugs on various systems or organs of the body
- Use of purgatives
- Administration of drugs dealing especially with:
  - dosage and timings
  - modes of administrating drugs

- forms and shapes of drugs

- Correction of harmful effects of drugs
- Drug substitutes.

Iranian pharmacology is very much concerned with the classification of drugs. Drugs in major are classified into four groups according to their qualities:

- drugs with Hot temperament
- drugs with cold temperament
- moist drugs (including lubricants)
- dry drugs

However, the most well-known classification is the distinction between simple (mofradat) and compound drugs (morakabat). 'Simples' are those drugs which occur in their natural and simple state. 'Compounds' are drugs as they are usually understood today. The branch of Iranian pharmacology dealing with compounds is usually discussed under the topic of *gharabadin* which means drugs catalogue, pharmacopoeia, or medical formulary.

It is important that the full significance of Iranian pharmacology be made better known to the modern world, especially in the light of the threat to human health posed by many synthetic or chemical drugs.

Manipulative techniques

In Persian Medicine, manipulative techniques are not usually approved unless it is considered absolutely essential. It is generally considered that manipulative techniques were limited to the various forms of cauterization, massage, venesection etc. It is also referred that osteology, which is still widely practiced today in many parts of the world.

In Persian Medicine naturally grown herbs are generally used according to their temperament in various types of ailments. Use of mineral and animal drugs is also made following the specific treatment methodology (like purgation etc.) and temperamental expression of the patient. It is interesting to note that the many physicians encouraged poly-pharmacy and amassed a large number of pharmaceutical remedies. However, with the process of the revival of /alternative medicines all over the globe, once again use of simples is being promoted and work on preparation of lists of essential herbal drugs on regional and international level is underway.

Diagnosis

In the Persian Medicine, diagnosis is made on the basis of clinical observations of the patients. For instance, finding the conjunctiva yellow, the diagnosis is made as jaundice. In this way for diagnosing a disease, physical observations are the principal guidelines in this system.

The observations are based on the following points:

- History of the patient - present and past along with family history

- External signs visible by the naked eye and also by touch sensation

- Pulse

- Urine

- Stool

Treatment

In the Persian Medicine the patient is treated by:

- Herbs (mostly in crude form, their parts or as a whole)

▪ Animal products (substances derived from animals such as amber, castoreum, corals, honey, canthridium, pearls etc.)

▪ Minerals (such as ammonium chloride, arsenic, asphalt, bole armeniac, potassium carbonate, borax, silver foil, soapstone etc.)

Generally, the drugs used are based on poly-pharmacy but the use of simples is also prevalent. Some recent studies are being conducted to rationalize a list of "Essential Herbal Drugs" which can be used without any fear of side effects round the globe for all age groups in recommended doses. The medicines can be used in the form of: aqua distillates, syrups, extracts, powders, pills/tablets, infusions, decoctions, electuary, oils, resins, fermented compounds, dentifrices, collyriums, calcined preparations, itrifals, preserves, confections, pastes, etc.

Prescriptions of the drugs for various treatments are generally based on:

▪ Temperament of the patient and state of the disease,

▪ Pharmacological activities and temperamental attribute (properties) of drugs,

▪ The possible form in which the drugs (simple/compound) may be used.

Prescriptions began with the legend Allah is the Healer. These contain information about the dosage and how to prepare a specific medicine. Medicine is usually prescribed initially for some days; treatment being continued or changed according to the response of the patient. Diet is also prescribed accordingly. Medicines are prescribed considering the following points:

(a) Sex,

(b) Age,

(c) Habits,

(d) Climate and time,

(e) Atmosphere (environment) of the patient and his creed,

(f) Power (immunity) of the patients,

(g) Temperament,

(h) Body Structure,

(i) Major Symptoms,

(j) Psychology,

(k) Patient's view about time of crisis he/she is facing,

(I) accompanying complaints along with actual disease,

(m) Condition of Stomach,

(n) Idiosyncrasy,

(o) Route of drugs,

(p) Major and minor pharmacological actions of drugs,

(q) Outcome/effects/side effects of medicines used previously

(r) Occupation and earnings. In case of emergencies, specific treatment is given or advised according to the situation.

The human body is given due respect and treated as a 'whole', so the treatment varies with the condition of patient and the state of the disease. In the first instance

(1) Nutrition or nutritional treatment is advised. In the 2nd stage (2) Nutritional medicines are prescribed. In the 3rd stage Medicines which also have nutritional attributes are given. In the 4th stage (4) Medicines which have desired activity are administered.

Treatment also includes: Anti-pathogenic treatment and systematic general treatment (where herbs of low potency are used).

Elements (Philosophical Concept)

Many philosophies and worldviews have a set of classical elements believed to reflect the simplest essential parts and principles of which anything consists or upon which the constitution and fundamental powers of anything are based. Most frequently, classical elements refer to ancient beliefs inspired by natural observation of the phases of matter; with the classical elements: earth is equivalent to solid, water is equivalent to liquid, air is equivalent to gas and fire is equivalent to plasma. Elements are not the real fire, air, water and earth, but these are the four states of matter described in terms of physical attributes as cosmological factors.

The elements are defined by Persian Medicine system of medicine as:

Elements are simple indivisible matters which provide the primary components for the human body and other lively substances. They cannot be further resolved into simpler entities. The various substances (compounds) in the nature depend upon these elements for their existence on their intermixture (specific chemical combinations) (Avicenna 980-1037 A.D.)

The modern definition of elements is yet more simplified. It states; by the term element is meant constituents of substances which cannot be further separated qualitatively.

Thus, the account of elements given by Avicenna fully satisfies that there is hardly any difference between the ancient and modern concepts of elements. The difference, however, is in the approach for the elements described by Avicenna encircle the wide view of cosmological (in terms philosophical) factors, whereas the modern view is limited being materialistic and restricted to the periodic table. Cosmic elements are those from which animals, plants and stones, all are ulimately made of.

Scientists and philosophers believed such elements to be four: Air, water, earth and fire, and have the qualities of these elements, moisture, cold, dryness and heat in varying proportions.

Avicenna claims that elements are simple indivisible matters (qualitatively - which lose their desired activities on disintegration or acquire new ones on combination addition with other elements) which provide primary components for the living beings and other substances of the universe. They cannot be further resolved into simpler entities and the various substances (compounds) in nature depend for their existence on their intermixture (i.e. the chemical combinations). Avicenna says that it is but essential for a physician to admit that elements are neither more than four in number, nor less than four and among them fire and air are lighter and earth and water are heavier (canon of medicine).

In Persian Medicine, contrary to the modern concept of cell, the lowest level of human body organization and other living creations is the element. About 2500 years back the ancient Greek scholar Democritus and his pupil who introduced the idea that all matters were made up of small indivisible units called Atoma (atoms). Today we are aware of the fact that the atoms are combined in different ways to yield monomers (amino acids, nucleotides, monosaccharaides etc.) which are the building blocks of biological macromolecules (peptides, nucleic acids, polysaccharides etc.)

The constituents of our humors

Further, the macromolecules are combined with smaller molecules to form cell organelles (the constituent parts of rotoobat-e-gharizi) i.e. cell-membrane, mitochondria, endoplasmic reticulum and lysosomes etc. The organelles are combined to form cells, the cells to form tissues, the tissues to form organs; and organs to form organism. Thus, instead of starting study of human body from the level of a cell, the physicians begin their study from the very lowest level of organization i.e. elements (and atoms). This approach has its own significance from the following points of view;

Creation of individual by the Lord of the Universe Who produced the shape of man by clay and water, solidified (made it light) it over fire by (maturation/concoction) and entered air (spirit) in its body.

Elements are among the principles and have been taken from the physical sciences as such, and the essential (basic) or the primary elemental compositions like amino acids, hormones, enzymes, vitamins and active principles of plants - all true natural combinations each being complete individual structural units under Avicenna's definition (of elements) are considered as elements of today's functional and theoretical science. Study of all active elements is being conducted under a newly emerging science of Elementology.

Philosophical Overview of Four- Elements

Human body, just like everything else in the universe, according to Persian Medicine, is composed of four elements, earth, water, air and fire. Earth represents solids, water the liquids, air the gases and fire the heat (or energy) of the body. Exponents of this theory hold that these four elements contribute to the formation of things in nature, had there been only one element, the living body should never have disintegrated from any (external) adverse influence.

The concept was widely accepted and in fact all other followers of Avicenna belonging to pedestrians became exponent of this concept and consequently Persian Medicine was incarcerated in the dilemma of fours. They attributed binary qualities to each of the 'element' to express its temperamental state (specific humoral dominance) and exhibiting physical properties. These are as follows:

(Fire)-Hot and Dry

(Air)-Hot and Moist

(Water)-Cold and Moist

(Earth)-Cold and Dry

In fact, the above four elements are four states of matter and can be described as follows;

Earth

A simple, solid element regarded as being normally situated in the center of other elements. On account of its absolute heaviness, it has a natural tendency to remain stationary unless it is away from its center (of gravity) when it (tends) to return to its (original) position.

In temperament it is so cold and dry that in the absence of external factors, its natural quality is readily perceived by the body. In nature its elemental character serves the purpose of making the compounds (objects) firm, stable, and lasting.

Water

A simple liquid substance which in its natural state surrounds the earth and in turn is engulfed by the air in its natural state or position. It is this relationship which accounts for its relatively heavy weight (for gravity).

Water is cold and moist, that is, in its pure and natural state it displays an obvious coldness and the quality of moisture. Moisture is the quality which makes it capable of ready dispersion and aggregation and which enables it to accept varied shapes of an unstable kind.

Air

A simple gaseous element whose natural position is above other elements being higher than even the atmosphere of the earth. This is known as its absolute lightness.

It is the macrocosmic celestial element which is Hot and moist in nature and corresponds within the microcosmic interpretation as blood.

Fire

A simple energy bearing Hot and dry element necessary for the proper maturation of constituents and for making them light. Combined with other elements, it facilitates the diffusion of air, attenuates the coldness and heaviness of the earth and water by imparting them its own elemental qualities which are opposed to those of their own (particularly) temperament.

Fire being a form of energy was included later in the list of basic elements because of the ancient philosophers who observed that without fire (heat) the very existence of life is impossible. Each and every chemical reaction whether inorganic or organic, through which large molecules are formed (Anabolism) or from which small ones are formed (Catabolism) requires the presence of heat (certain degree of temperature) i.e. either the energy is taken in or given out. Likewise, in the human body, formation of compounds or their break-up into smaller units (viz. the elements) is not possible unless that is provided. In addition to this, the law of transformation of energy reveals that fire is another form of matter (elements).

Universal Distribution of Elements

Now keeping in view the periodic table, more than one hundred elements have been discovered and their physical, chemical (and of many) biochemical properties have been discovered. These elements could well be classified according to their physical and chemical properties in four groups (cosmic/philosophic/states of matter). Some of them are solids, some liquids, some in gaseous state and some fiery - highly combustible for prune to react very hastily and actively with other elements to form new compounds. Furthermore, when some elements are transformed into energy i.e. fire, it becomes another state of matter.

Human Elements

About nineteen of the elements participate into the elementary composition of human body. The six basic elements; oxygen, carbon, hydrogen, nitrogen, phosphorus and sulphur contribute to about 97% of the total cell mass of living organisms and provide the structural element to the protoplasm (rotoobat-e-gharizi). The metallic elements including sodium, potassium, calcium, copper, zinc, selenium, silicon, molybdenum, fluorine, chlorine, iodine, manganese, cobalt, iron are considered to contribute about 3% for the cell.

While some of them provide structural element to the protoplasm of the cells, the others (like trace elements) remain in their elemental or other forms (in hormones, enzymes, amino acids etc.) in the cell or in physiological system, run through the help of body fluids (humors) and play their roles in health and disease situations accordingly.

Specific (Chemical) Forms of Elements

Avicenna's theory holds that the chemical properties of elements depend upon their specific forms (e.g. the groups and classes of the periodic table). This specific chemical form (soorat-e-noeeye) is that property of the substance which determines its "internal structure" which is specific for that particular substance. Any change in its chemical form results a change (or disruption) in its chemical, and thereby its biochemical and physiological properties. Therefore, when we interpret this hypothesis on chemical elements (of periodic table) we understand that the chemical (specific) form of an element is nothing but its atomic structure that depends upon the atomic number. No two elements carry the same atomic number, but the atomic weights may be the same (Isobars). When two (or more) elements have the same atomic number but different atomic weight these are known as Isotopes. Similarly, the specific chemical form of a compound depends upon the molecular structure of that compound. Therefore, any change in the molecular structure results a change in its chemical properties i.e. the compound is changed into another compound.

Qualities and Characteristics of Elements

Qualities and characteristics of elements according to Persian Medicineare described in terms of their temperament which is expressed in terms of their duplex qualities among the four; these are Hot (hot) and cold, moistness (wet) or dry. Heat and cold are considered as active qualities and moistness and dryness as passive qualities. According to the theory of opposites, generally two non-antagonistic properties are combined together to express specific temperament of a body, be it human, animal, plant or other living organisms.

However, it should be borne in mind that when the ancient philosophers say anything Hot, cold, moist or dry, they generally referred to one of the following three meanings.

١ Somtímes a thing which is called Hot or cold is actually (functionally) Hot or cold i.e. When it is touched it feels actually Hot or cold.

٢ Somtimes a thing which is said to be Hot or cold is not actually Hot or cold and does not feel actually Hot or cold on touching, but it is potentially Hot or cold i.e. When it enters into the body it produces heat or raises the temperature, or reduces the production of heat or lowers the body temperature. The similar case is with the moist and dry things too.

Somtimes a thing which is said to be Hot or cold, or moist or dry is neither actually nor potentially Hot, cold, moist or dry, but it carries some symbolic meaning, just like charm, color or flavor for quark are arbitrarily fixed by modern physicists which have no relationship with the actual meanings of these words. Thus a substance is said to be Hot when after entering into the body it shows certain subjective and objective symptoms which are arbitrarily fixed for the intense biological reaction. This also holds good to other qualities i.e. cold, moist and dry.

From the foregoing account it may be evident that elements are not only four in numbers but there are four categories of elements based on four states of biological, biochemical, biomedical manifestation of elements. Moreover, from the definition of elements given by Avicenna it is evident that the substances which are simple (mofrad) could only be included in the list of elements, and if any substance which was earlier considered as element due to researches and by experiments, and now due to availability of elaborate methods of laboratory tests and isolation, the same has been found as compound; then we must refer to the concept of exhibiting specific temperament and specific composition by elements, and specific activity being rendered by specific compounds as we have studied under the heading of specific chemical forms (soorat-e-noeeye). Now, in this broad context as each element for treating living beings has been accorded specific temperament (the plants, plant parts, minerals, animal parts, insects etc.) by Iranian physicians.

therefore (as principal) each can be treated as simple (mofrad) and the continuously explored chemical compounds (of biological significance) like vitamins, enzymes, hormones and other active principles or ingredients can be regarded as constituting or physiologically active elements of an individual element. Thus it is true to say that research from the modern point of view is retrogressive, because we are emphasizing upon the lowest unit which constitutes an organism, substance or individual. Whereas the Iranian scholars, scientists and philosophers though identified the importance of units, they did not deviate from the ideology of ascribing four-elements-qualities to each of the element described or present on the mother earth. Thus the words like; Simple=Single=Unit=Element can be regarded as synonyms. This might be one of the reasons that physicians of Iranian Materia Medica call their texts of Persian Medicines as Compendium or Book of Simples (mofradat book).

Avicennahas himself advised that it is necessary for a physician to accept elements from natural philosophy. Therefore, it is imperative for us to accept his teachings and hence, accept the number of arkan given by the present *tabiyat (Physis),* the natural philosophy of today. A curious fact should also be accepted that if the number of elements given by modern science is accepted in place of four elements, we would certainly find that it would make no difference to our basic concepts, because we would be presenting the concept of elements in its correct perspective. And thus it would be a great service to Persian Medicine instead of rendering any harm to it.

Furthermore, this fact should also be admitted that significance of arkan is not only limited to their study as structural and functional units of our body but they also influence our body in many other ways and they play an immense role in the diagnosis and treatment of disease too.

Humors (Structural Components)

Humors are defined as the structural components of the body, are composed of elements and natures in different mixtures, proportions and combinations. These are supposed to constitute building units of organs and thus, body, and are considered as primary body fluids produced from digested food.

The Persian Medicine postulates the presence of four Humors in the body. They are: phlegm, blood, yellow bile and black bile, corresponding to the four elements and their four primary qualities. The basis of this postulation is the separation from blood (under various circumstances) of substances having these four humoral attributes. When these Humors are present in the right proportion in a body, the body is healthy; when this proportion is disturbed, loss of health may result. In order to restore health, it is necessary to restore the balance of Humors. These (four) Humors are also referred as the real fluids (rotoobat-e-asli).

The concept of Humors has occupied a central place in Persian Medicine. It is one of the seven basic physiological principles (omoor-e-tabieeye). It belongs to those basic concepts of Persian Medicine which include the distinguishing features of this unique healing art. It is a system developed by our physicians to explain all physiological and pathological processes in the human body in terms of body fluids.

The word Humors is a Persian Medicine term which literally stands for admixture (humor). But in Persian Medicine terms all fluids of the body (roboobat-e-badani) are called Humors owing to the fact that the fluids of the body are not a single entity but are intermixed with each other especially in the blood vessels, these are of different types and properties and serve different functions. Therefore, these are called as Humors. Keeping in view the diverse properties and functions of Humors, the following definition seems to be more appropriate.

"Humors are those moist and fluid parts of the body which are produced after transformation ofspecific form (soorat-e-noeeye), and metabolism of the elements, they serve the function of nutrition, growth and repair; and produce energy for the preservation of individual and his species. A right proportion and intermixture (homeostasis/proper balance) of them, according to quantity and quality constitutes health, and disturbed or abnormal proportion or imbalance (dystemperament) according to quantity and quality, and irregular distribution leads to disease".

This humoral theory was postulated by Hippocrates in his book ***human nature*** as under:

"The body contains four (major kinds of) Humors, *blood, phlegm, yellow bile and black bile*; a right proportion, according to quality and quantity, and mixing of which (homoeostasis) constitutes health, and disproportion and irregular distribution, according to their quantity and quality constitutes disease".

Ali ibn-e-Abbas-e-Majusi ahvazi in his book Kamel al-Sana'at al-tebbiya has given a bit detailed account. He says:

▪ The basis of health is the right proportion and specific equilibrium of Humors according to their quality i.e. homoeostasis in the internal environment is maintained, the body remains healthy. Because the temperament of the internal environment remains normal. This is the basis of health and preventive medicine.

▪ That when the normal proportion and specific equilibrium of Humors is altered, the temperament (specific predominant state or homoeostasis) of the internal environment is imbalanced, and thus the disease is developed. This is the basis of etiology and pathology of disease.

- That when this wrong proportion and altered equilibrium of Humors i.e. imbalanced temperament is corrected, the health can be restored. This is the basis of treatment. Thus, the humoral theory deals with all the aspects of disease viz. etiology, pathology, prevention and treatment of the diseases, and, this holds good especially for metabolic and infectious diseases.

Application of the term humors on all the fluids of the body

All fluids of the body, without any exception are called as Humors. This can be proved by the following facts:

That the human body is composed of three kinds of things:

- The ***solid parts*** are known as organs of members which keep in their enclosure the two other parts, liquids and gases.

- The liquid parts are known as real fluids.

- The gaseous parts are known as ***pneuma or vital spirits*** (arvah).

The last two (B, C) things are being enclosed within the species of the organs.

The ***real fluids*** are of four kinds:

From the above account it is clearly evident that real fluids and Humors are synonymous and both stand for *blood, yellow bile, phlegm and black bile.*

Abu Sahl Masihi (died 999 AD.) the teacher of Avicenna also held the same views and says in his book that the entire body consists of three kinds of substances:

First among them are those which possess receptivity and hardness and do not, therefore, require to be enclosed in vessels to prevent them from flow. These are known as *organs.* Second are those which are moist and fluid substances enclosed in the vessels and (interstitial) spaces and cavities of the organs to prevent those (vessels) from flow. These are known as *Humors*, and the third are those which are gaseous and vapors, and are enclosed in hard vessels to prevent them from rapid diffusion. These are known as *pneuma.*

Thus, the solid part of the body is known as organs, fluid part is known as Humors and gaseous part is known as pneuma, and there is nothing of any other kind in the body. Hence, the term Humors is applicable to all fluids of the body, with no exception at all.

Likewise, Abu Sahl Masihi has classified *fevers* in three categories based on organs, Humors and pneuma. Here also he has included all fluids of the body in humor. He categorically says; there is nothing in the body which can be its component part except organs, Humors and pneuma/air. He therefore says that the subjects of *fevers* are either:

- organs which enclose fluids,

- Fluids which are being enclosed by the organs, or

- Pneuma which are diffused (into the organs and fluids of the body).

Thus, from the above mentioned statement it is fully evident that Abu Sahl Masihi gives no difference between *Humors and fluids*. Therefore, he included all fluids of the body in *Humors*.

Avicenna has (also) contended that the body is composed of only three parts viz. organs, fluids, and pneuma, and there is nothing of any sort except these components of the body. Thus he also classifies fevers in three categories according to (these) three component parts of the body.

- Hectic fever, related to organs-tissues.

- Humoral fever related to Humors.

▪ Ephemeral fever related to pneuma/air.

Avicenna has (also) used the terms fluid and humors as synonymous. Thus, while dividing the body in its component parts he has used the term fluids and where he has signified this with fever he has used the term Humors.

Aghili khorasani also maintain that all fluids of the body are humors. Thus, from the preceding account following inference can be derived.

▪ The term Humors is applicable to all fluids of the body irrespective of their color, location, quantity and quality (composition). And therefore, intracellular fluids (rotoobat-e-ostoghosi), intercellular or tissue fluids and trans-cellular fluids (rotoobat-e-tajavif), and vascular fluids (rotoobat-e-orooghi) are called asHumors. All electrolytes and organic compounds constituting these Humors whether they are proteins, lipids, and carbohydrates according to their chemical nature (soorat-e-noeeye) or they are enzymes, hormones or vitamins according to their physiological function; whether they are in elemental or otherwise, in their compound states; whether they are acidic, basic or neutral; whether they are crystalloids or colloids, or they carry any electrical charge or are neutral, determine the qualityof Humors as their component parts.

▪ That Humors are not only four in numbers but phlegm, blood, yellow bile and black bile, are four *major divisions* which can be subjected to further subdivisions: and thus the number of Humors reaches to hundreds or thousands.

Origin of humors

The Four Humors are responsible for the nutrition, growth and metabolism of the organism. They originate in the digestive process.

In Persian Medicine, digestion happens in four stages:

The First Digestion happens in the gastrointestinal tract, and produces chyle; its waste product is the feces, or stool.

The Second Digestion happens in the liver, and produces the Four Humors. Its wastes are eliminated via the bile, urine and sweat.

The Third Digestion happens in the blood vessels, and feeds the principal organs of the body. Its wastes are eliminated via the sweat.

The Fourth Digestion happens in the tissues, and is the final congelation of the Four Humors into living tissue. Its wastes are eliminated similarly to the Third Digestion.
The Four Humors originate in the liver in the Second Digestion as follows:

Blood, or the Sanguine humor, is the first to arise, and receives the richest, choicest share of nutrients. It is the most plentiful humor, and enters the general circulation.

Phlegm, as Plasma or the Phlegmatic humor is the second to arise and receives the next richest share of nutrients. It is also very plentiful, and enters the general circulation.
Yellow Bile, or the Choleric humor, is the third to arise and receives a rather coarse, meager share of nutrients. It is not so plentiful. Only a slight residue enters the general circulation; the rest is stored in the gall bladder, its receptacle, to be used as needed.

Black Bile, or the Melancholic humor, is the last to arise, and receives the coarsest, most meager share of nutrients. It is the least plentiful. Only a slight residue enters the general circulation; the rest is stored in the spleen, its receptacle, to be used as needed. The first two humors, blood and phlegm, are moist and flourishing, and are the metabolic agents of the Wet elements - Air and Water, respectively. Most of the nutrition, growth and metabolism of the organism depend on them.

The last two humors, yellow bile and black bile, are dry and effete, and only needed by the organism in small amounts. They are the metabolic agents of the Dry elements - Fire and Earth, respectively. Although only needed in small amounts, they are potent and essential catalysts where needed.

Characteristic features of the four Humors:

- Blood is red in color and Hot and moist in nature. It provides nourishment to the body and acts as fuel to the human body as well as generates heat. Blood is of two kinds: normal and abnormal. Normal blood is red in color, has a sweet taste and no abnormal odor. Locus of blood is considered to be the liver.

- Phlegm is (fluid) whitish in color, and is cold and moist in nature. It is capable of being converted into blood. It provides nourishment to the brain, lubricates the joints, and keeps the tissues and organs of the body moist. Depending upon taste and consistency it has many abnormal forms. No special location, identified as the part of non-nutritious residue rejected by the physiological process of digestion.

- Yellow bile which is Hot and dry in nature occurs in normal as well as abnormal forms. Normally, it is bright saffron-red and is light and pungent. Its function is to attenuate the blood so that it reaches the minute channels of the body. It nourishes the lungs, cleanses the walls of the bowels and stimulations them. Locus of yellow bile is said to be the gall bladder.

- Black bile forms the sediment of the blood and provides nourishment to bones and in the stomach stimulations appetite. Locus of black bile is referred to be the spleen.

Predominance of a particular humor

(Specific Temperamental State of Individuals)

Based upon the predominance of a particular humor in an Individual, four types of personalities are described:

▪ The sanguine type: Such individuals are obese and possess Hot and moist qualities. They are active, have a good appetite and a full strong pulse. Their complexion is reddish and they pass reddish-tinged urine.

▪ The bilious or choleric type: These individuals are lean and hairy, have sallow sclera of the eyes, and a sallow complexion in general. They get angry quickly and possess Hot and dry features. They are energetic and clever and have strong sexual desires. They have prominent blood vessels and a strong, rapid pulse. They pass yellowish-colored urine.

▪ The phlegmatic type: Such individuals are obese and flaccid with whitish skin. They possess cold and moist attributes. Their hair is thin and their blood vessels are hardly visible through the skin. They are sluggish in walk and intellect and are not inclined much towards sex or hunger. Their urine is colorless and they are hardly ever thirsty.

▪ The melancholic type: They are thin, dark with narrow blood vessels and slow pulse. By nature, they are cold and dry. They have only a slight sexual urge and suffer from sleeplessness. Their urine is mixed with a tinge of reddish green.

State of Dominance of a Humor

▪ If among the Humors, the blood carries dominance, sleep and migraine are exaggerated, vessels turgid and red, Somtimes thought revolts; there is a heaviness of the head, weakness of sensation, carelessness, Hotth to the touch, heaviness of the shoulders, yawning; Somtimes heaviness of the flanks; nose bleeding, the desire to stretch out, relaxing of the abdomen, search for a life of well-being, dreams, varied joys, and of all colors, gaiety, longing for phlebotomy, unusual ruddiness of the eyes, furuncles and pustules, dreams of sweet things, a sugar flavor in the mouth, as if the patient had just eaten some. If these symptoms are seen in the spring or during the prime of youth, they indicate diseases of the blood.

▪ If bile is dominant, the shade of the body is yellow, the appetite weak, and the mouth bitter. There is gastric burning, vomiting of bile, a severe diarrhea, restlessness, sunken eyes, dry mouth, and tongue. At times, the urine is yellow, the patient has episodes of syncope, some goose-bumps, is sad, is thirsty without appetite, and dreams of flames; his Pulse is weak, his body febrile. Frequent Hot baths are the cause of this state as are sojourns in southern countries, and prolonged misuse of spiced food, especially in the summer.

▪ If black bile dominates, the body is Hot, thoughts sullen, appetite reduced, an acid flavor in the mouth. On examination, anguish rigidness of the face, pulse firm in its slowness; the patient is constipated, presents black spots, sadness, restlessness, without agitation. The urine is white, not very dense, and crude; similarly, the stools are not digested. The causes are dry food, anxiety, permanent sadness and misery. In his dreams, the patient sees dangers and completely frightening things. This affects the mature age in autumn, in northern countries and the weakened individuals.

▪ Phlegm dominates, the head is heavy, the sleep prolonged, there is a laziness of movements, little appetite; plethora is in harmony with the force of individual; he is slow in his gait, his intelligence is slow, he leans towards an unusual softness, foams, has a swollen face, his shade is dull; the pulse is slow and thick; urine dense, strong and crude; thirst is reduced except when phlegm is salty or decayed. Cause of this state is cold and moist food, old age, cold effects of season, sedentary, lack of Hot baths, Somtimes gluttony, the sojourn in a country because of its water flow; in his sleep the phlegmatic person dreams of seas, complains of nightmares and his chyme is not digested well.

The theory of four Humors had a most prolonged influence on medical thought and it illustrated most graphically the philosophical interpretation of disease. The humoral theory was the result of many brilliant and correct observations. It was logical, explained many phenomena of health and disease, and gave valuable guidance to the medical practitioners and it was not scientific in our sense of the word: nobody had even seen the black bile and the qualities Hot, cold, dry, moist were not physical concepts.

Scientific experiments have been conducted in biology too, but the scientific means (as to explain or observe Humors in physical sense) were not available for an interpretation of health and disease, and the need for a comprehension of these phenomena was satisfied by philosophic speculation.

Classification of Humors

- According to their locations.
- According to their color.
- According to their body needs

o(Excrementitiously/ Non- excrementitiously)

oGood humors- Normal

oBad humors, Normal - no physical function

oWaste humors (redundant humor)

oThe above mentioned three types of humors are specific for individual types of cells and tissues, they articulate to form specialized organs and to assist their physiological function. Their volume and consistency in terms of biochemical analysis are indicators for disease states i.e. they provide means of laboratory diagnosis. The following three (D, E, F) humors are also important from the standpoint of philosophy but seem to compromiseadvanced classified groups e.g. Primary/Secondary, Fine/Coarse and Normal/Abnormal.

- According to their conditions: Primary /Secondary Encircled fluid type, interstitial fluids, Congealed fluids, Seminal fluid
- According to their qualities – fineness/coarseness

- According to their nature i.e. normal and abnormal.

Classification of humors according to Location:

- Stout fluid
- Vascular fluid
- Cavities fluid

- **Stout fluid:** It is the humor responsible for binding the organs together. Contained within the cells it may be identified as the intracellular fluid (or protoplasm) of the cell, which is the unit of tissues. This humor is supposed to establish the internal environment of the cells, and the normal temperament/quality or homeostasis of each type of cells depends upon specific predominant type of humor. This humor is also called real fluid, instinctive fluid or pristine fluid.

- **Vascular fluid:** Contained within the vessels (either veins or arteries), for example the blood (and the bile). It is also among the real fluid/pristine fluid.

- **Cavities fluid:** Contained within the spaces between the cells, the tissue spaces and various cavities of the body. This humor thus may be identified as the tissue fluid, intercellular fluid and trans-cellular fluid. This fluid establishes communication between real fluid (intracellular fluid) and the internal environment of the body, and temperament (homoeostasis) in the internal environment depends upon the quantity and quality of this humor.

Above mentioned are the most common (generally identified) types of humors, however there are many other need scientific interpretation and which are formed during the course of the completion of physiological phenomena.

Classification of humors according to Color:

Comprehensively it must be borne in mind that on the basis of color there are four major divisions of humors:

- Red: blood,

- White: phlegm

- Yellow: yellow bile,

- Black: black bile

Sub-divisions of above mentioned (parent) humors on the basis of color can be made as following:

- All the colorless (or white) fluids of the body, irrespective of their locations are called as phlegm.

- All the fluids of the body which are yellow in color are called as yellow bile.

- All those fluids of the body which are blue, brown or black in color are identified as black bile.

- All the fluids of the body which are red or tend to become red are known as blood.

Theory of Humors asserts that *'blood'* is admixture of all the above kinds of humors and all these may be found in blood. In other words, blood is the name of admixture of all humors (in the body). Places or the organs from where specific humors produce or reside, all of these are present in requisite proportion in the blood in an individual, constitute the specific humoral composition, with specific predominance (of a humor) and thus specific temperament of an individual.

Classification of humors according to their Body Needs:

There are two such (major) kinds:

▪ good Humors: Produced in the body in normal way, are always needed by the body and serve specific physiological functions, for example:

Normal blood and its constituents

Normal bile

Normal phlegm

Normal black bile

These good humors are therefore also known as normal or non-excrementitiously Humors.

▪ Bad Humors: Produced normally in the course of metabolism but do not serve any specific physiological function and therefore are needed to be expelled out of the body (excrements, excreta, waste products or excrementitiously Humors) for example: urine, stool, menstrual blood.

These excrementitiously Humors are also known as waste humor (khelt-e-radi).

According to Avicenna, good humor (alone or in combined form) possesses the property of becoming part of an organ or attaining (or developing into) shape of an organ when the body needs or possesses the capability to replace the wear and tear of an organ, whereas waste humor has no property of becoming the part of the body. Exception of becoming a valid humor for body by this type of humor is the case when whole of this humor is completely expelled out of the body and then after reentrance or reformation it may acquire the form of good humor.

Classification of humors according to their Conditions:

Avicenna has divided all fluids of the body into two kinds:

a) primary fluids

b) Secondary fluids

▪ *Primary fluids* are those very four humors which circulate within the blood vessels are called as primary fluids.

▪ *Secondary fluids* include all those fluids of the body which are converted from primary condition to secondary and have diffused into the organs (cell ► tissue organization) but they have not become the part of tissue - cells practically. Such fluids are four in number:

▪ The encircled fluid.

▪ The interstitial fluid.

▪ The nearly congealed fluid.

▪ The seminal fluid.

These fluids are considered as those which have passed from blood vessels (capillaries) to tissues and cells and have transformed into various stages and forms. With the exceptions of few physicians of Persian Medicine all categorically mention and amply prove Secondary fluids (being fluids) as types of humors.

Classification of humors according to their Quality:

There are two such types:

▪ *Fine Humors*: Those fluids or parts of fluids (Humors) which have the property of diffusing into cells and tissues and when they combine with *pneuma*, they produce *energy* to perform various physiological functions in the body.

▪ *Coarse/Turbid Humors*: Those fluids or parts of fluids (Humors) which perform the function of *anabolism* and become part of the organs. They replace wear and tear and promote growth.

Classification of humors according to their Nature:

There are two types of humors according to their nature:

- *Normal humors*: When the primary or secondary humors and other fluids e.g. given under *real fluid* or different kinds of humors are categorized according to their locations are normal with reference to their *quantity* and *quality* are called as normal humors, for example normal blood, normal bile, normal cerebrospinal fluid, normal synovial fluid, normal chyme etc.

- *Abnormal humors*: When the quality and composition of normal humors is altered due to any cause, its behavioral pattern (in physiology or action) or *temperament* is altered. Hence it is called as abnormal. For example, black bile is found in normal state in the body but when there is any alteration or indifference in its composition and quantity is caused it, turns into *atrabilious*, this is the abnormal black bile.

Such abnormalities in humors (Humors/body fluids) take place in two ways:

- Any humor itself becomes altered, thereby its quality and temperament within the body is changed. There are lot many causes which correlate with the symptoms in specific (ailment) conditions.

- Any humor is mixed with another normal or abnormal humor and owing to this (mixture), its normal temperament is altered. This may also happen due to various causes.

Temperament (Behavioural Components)

Temperament (according to Persian Medicine) is defined as the pattern of activity and reactivity in living beings, in natural articles, substances or their parts used as drugs or medicines. The heat (Hot) and cold in drugs may be identified with the dispersive and aggregative aspects of energy, while moisture and dryness with the receptive and resistant aspects of mass respectively.

Since the four primary qualities of elements (being Hot, cold, dryness and moisture) neither entirely absent from the constitution of any object, nor are they present in absolutely equal proportion, their interaction produces specific predominance of a (humoral) constitution like finger-prints of an individual or unique of any particular object (due to specific elementary physical/physico-chemical attributes).

Theoretically, temperament is of two kinds:

- Balanced When the opposing qualities of the temperament (formed) are quantitatively exactly equal and the balance is an absolute average of these qualities, and

- Imbalanced when the qualities of the temperament (formed) are unequal and inclined towards one side.

Temperament is expressed by the Persian Medicine concepts of its being sanguine, phlegmatic, choleric or melancholic according to the respective preponderance of the Humors. Interpreted in modern terminology it is the specific constitution of an individual's psycho-neuro-endocrinal system with its orientation tempered different in each individual.

Temperament of Drugs and Medicines

Natural drugs being composite units and being simple or compoun in formulation are also assigned temperaments but drugs are classified under four physical orders (of temperament viz. first, second, third and fourth). Temperaments of drugs are identified in relation with their elementological physical actions which they exert on the human body. Thus a drug is said to be Hot means that, when it enters the body and interact with the vital faculties, it produces (temperamental) effect which is Hot. Drugs are principally used to improve the health state, correct the abnormal physiological or pathological (humoral imbalanced) states of the body or any particular system, process or disease-state of an organ.

Some definitions

Normal drugs

According to Avicenna, When the physicians mention about a drug that is normal or balanced, neither they mean to state that the drug in fact is normal (in composition because no such body occurs on the earth where in its composition the four elements: fire, earth, water and air are in equal proportion), nor they mean that it has such balance as that of human individuals and or its temperament is like that of living beings. They actually mean that when such administered drugs interact with the vital force of the body and digestive power of the organs, they bring the active constituents out of the drug for relevant action, then such a constitutional condition is produced which remains within the temperamental limits of the individual thus normal/balanced drugs produce no such effect which in any way is deviated from the normal (temperament), and such drug due to its limited pharmacological action is regarded as normal/balanced.

Hot and Cold Drugs

Similarly, when it is mentioned by the Hakims about a drug that it is Hot or cold, it does not mean that its active constituent is Hot or cold in effect, nor it means that this Hot or cold attribute of drug in question is comparable to the individual. But it means that the referred drug produces as much Hotness or coldness within the body which is somewhat higher than the normal body coldness or Hotness. And as the finger-print phenomenon of temperament is different (specific) for each individual, therefore the degree or order of the pharmacological effect of drug varies for each individual up to certain extent. Hence, one drug can be extremely cold or hot for one individual and only cold or Hot for the other. It is the reason that when one drug does not produce desired action then it is advised to refer other drug of same order for an individual.

Establishing temperaments of drugs

Quantitative action or dose-related time-controlled experiments are necessary to establish temperament of natural drugs. Principles of such experiments include:

- Administration of the drug must be in recommended doses; it must not exceed the limits described.

- Administration must be in accordance with the prescription e.g. once, twice or thrice a day or as prescribed by the physician.

- Administration for experiment purpose must be done in a body with normal/balanced temperament.

- Administration for experiment must be done under normal climatic factors, temperature and time.

Thus, drugs which pass through such controlled experiments for the establishment of their temperament are afterwards assigned certain orders (First, Second, Third and Fourth Order Drugs).

Classification of drugs on the basis of temperament

As regards further classification, each order drugs have been sub-classified into three types:

Any Order, may be Hot/Cold, Dry/Moist in the said order

1st, 2nd, 3rd or 4th in the beginning (weak), middle (average) or in the end (potent).

Whereas,

Beginning: indicates the weaker action of drug in the said order,

Middle: indicates the average action of drug in the said order,

End: indicates the potent action of drug in the said order.

Classification of drugs can be simply shown in given table:

Normal/Balanced (Average Action) Drugs

Non-toxic; useful for all age groups in all seasons. Normal in at least two characteristics

First Order

Dose-related effects, repeatedly administered prescription drugs.

1(Weak Action)

2(Average Action)

3(Potent Action)

Second Order

Average group drugs Administered under prescription. Large doses administered repeatedly may cause harm to organs and general body constitution.

1(Weak Action)

2(Average Action)

3(Potent Action)

Third Order

Toxic Drugs, only administered under prescription. Potent drug of third order is considered as inclined towards poisonous group.

1(Weak Action)

2(Average Action)

3(Potent Action)

Fourth Order (Very Potent Action)

Poisonous Drugs

Thus drug belonging to third order in the end shall undoubtedly be toxic in action but shall be considered poisonous due to its inclination towards fourth order.

Small doses may cause fatality or exert deteriorative actions, only administered in threatened or lifesaving situations under physician's prescription in recommended doses (either detoxified or given with most appropriate corrigents).

As the table shows, to maintain a standard, drugs have been classified into certain orders due to their quick or slow and dose-related (well-known or desired) actions. Keeping in view their pharmacological action and effects, physicians have classified natural drugs into above four orders in addition to the normal/balanced order drugs.

First Order Drugs

The condition or effect produced by such drugs i.e. Hotness or coldness is not apparently perceived by the body or the relevant organ. However, if administered repeatedly then its actions (general or local) become evident. Action of first order drugs becomes also noticeable or apparent if these are administered in comparatively large doses.

Second Order Drugs

The condition or effect produced by such drugs is comparatively pronounced but not so much that could affect the organs' function. However, if there persists already an adverse or abnormal condition in the body (like tendency of diarrhea) then it may potentiate or substantiate such conditions. Repeated administration or in large doses but under prescription may bring desired change (affirmative or negative) in functions or may exert adverse effects on the organs.

Third Order Drugs

The condition or effect produced by such drugs due to their action and intensity is apparent or symptomatically detectable, but the damage or harm is not so grieving so as to cause fatality or produce acute toxicity. However, their repeated use or large doses administration is toxic, poisonous or fatal to the body.

Fourth Order Drugs (Toxic Drugs)

The condition or affect produced by such drugs due to their potentially toxic action is mostly harmful or adverse and their use is advised in small doses for short duration. Such drugs are either detoxified before use or used with the proper corrigent. Such drugs use is advised only in most essential disease states to evacuate the defined or well-identified pathological (mal humor) states that cannot be controlled or treated by above three order drugs. Difference between toxic and poisonous drugs is that, action of toxic drugs results into specific toxic condition (pharmacologically identified state) whereas, poisons' action proceed due to their molecular structures (which become the cause of adverse chemical changes in the body).

Modern interpretation in the light of elementology/ phytochemistry

As described in the beginning, drugs like other substances are characterized by their own physical qualities, but when in medicine a drug is termed hot, cold, dry or moist, it means that after its action and reaction in the body, it produces a perceptible degree of heat, cold, dryness or moisture in the body. Drugs are therefore graded from one to four orders and their respective types according to their dominant quality and are used to treat diseases of opposite qualities. Every substance has a temperament of its own. The basic qualities of energy being Hot and cold (opposite), and of mass being dryness and moisture, their mutual interaction lead to the emergence of a (new) balance of qualities which vary in quantitative proportion of the primary cosmic qualities (earth, fire, water and air).

Reflecting on the heating, cooling, dry and moist attributes of drugs in the sense as these are employed in Persian Medicine, a far wider basis for generalization might be arrived at as to the relationship between chemical constitution (composition) and (pharmacognostic) characteristics of drugs with reference to their pharmacological (mode of) action on human body is concerned.

We may find that:

- In case of drugs with significant constituents (alkaloid in character) containing a basic nitrogen atom are regarded as "Heating" and "Drying" in character.

- In case of drugs with significant constituent containing a carboxyl group (as in citrus, tamarind, unripe mango) are considered as "Cooling" in character.

- In case of drugs with significant constituent containing organically combined sulphur contribute towards the "Heating" attribute of a drug.

- In case of drugs like camphor where the significant constituent is a terpenic body is generally ascribed Cooling attributes.

There may be certain exceptions to such general concepts, as for instance opium is alkaloid in chemical nature but is considered to be cooling and glycyrrhiza with significant triterpenoid glycoside (glycyrrhizin) face confusion for being compound having opposite qualities (morakab-al-ghova), Hot and dry, or Hot and moist of first order. Problem of ascribing temperament therefore requires detailed study of the subsidiary constituents in so far as they may ulimately reveal the extent to which such variation and confusions may be due to them, or due to certain structural characteristics of the active constituents of the drug.

But whatever the case may be it is certain that phytochemistry and elementological composition seems valuable towards assigning particular temperament to individual plants, plant groups or products of natural origin.

The organs, the vital force, the bodily power and the corporeal functions

Organs, Vital Force, Bodily Powers and Corporeal Functions are the four working principles of body. Other major groups Elements, Humors and Temperaments have been discussed earlier. Theory of Persian Medicine holds that matter (may be individual or organic articles for biological use) in its different states and forms of existence helped by the humors (Humors the structural components of the body) produce specific temperament or the individual constitution. These structural components being continuously produced as a result of physiological processes combine to constitute the organs as well as the vital force (or the life-spirit). Organs equipped with the life spirit develop energy (Bodily Power) which is characterized by nature to manifest itself in Corporeal Functions (afaal) of a body or article. This group-wise classification hence embraces in it:

- the elementary constitution of the body (Elements)
- the structural components of the body (Humors)
- the physico-chemical constitution of the body(Temperaments)
- the anatomy of the body (Organs)
- the vital force of the body (pneuma /Life-force)
- the energy of the body (Energy)
- the physiology of the body (Physiological Functions/Actions)

This classification is in accordance with the accepted laws of science. The literature in Persian provides material for understanding each of them. These seven groups deal both with the normal and abnormal conditions. Knowledge of disease, etiology, pathology, semiology and therapeutics as well as of preventive medicine and infection are adequately dealt.

Organs

These are the simple or compound solid structures meant for carrying out specific or general functions for the body. Being essential members of the body are constituted from the coarser and solid particles of the structural components of Humors. The Masters of Persian Medicine say that Humors are the proximate principles for the human body. But the more proximate are cells and tissues and compound organs or mechanical organs.

Organs are divided into two major categories:

I: Simple organs cells and tissues.

II: Compound organs members of the body.

I: Simple Organs:

A simple organ is defined as the organ, smallest part of which exactly resembles the whole. A simple organ is therefore, homogeneous in structure throughout, e.g. a piece of bone. In fact, simple organs comprise tissues made up of primary combinations (i.e. combination of the smallest units of organs called cell). Though cell was not discovered as the simplest unit by the physicians and scientists but they were aware of the fact that simple organs are composed of some minute *matter* living unit capable of growth, movement and reproduction (cells) which were specific for each tissue (kind of cells).

In Persian Medicine is said:

"There is specific *matter* for each simple organ and there is specific form (soorat-e-noeeye), due to which it becomes specific species. This specific nature is common to the whole organ as well as any part of it. Owing to this, there is no difference between the whole and the part".

The bones, cartilages, ligaments and tendons, adipose, muscular and nervous tissues which support, interpret the functions of compound organs and protect them so that the whole body's form and constitution remains, maintained or kept in a balanced or perfect state.

Thus specific form of simple organ is actually the composition of its cells having specific form and character and become the basis of differentiation and distinction between different simple organs. Owing to this specific form one tissue differs from another in temperament and function.

II: Compound Organs:

A compound organ is defined as the organ which is composed of many simple organs/tissues and its constitution is heterogeneous. There are also known as the mechanical organs for example heart, liver, brain, stomach, hands, feet etc. Compound organs may be divided into four major types:

I: The Natural organs.

II: The Psychic or Mental organs.

III: The vital organs

IV: The Essential Vital organs.

I: The Natural Organs: Compound organs pertaining to natural faculty (ghova-e-tabiee) and natural functions (afaal-e-tabiee) are known as natural Organs (aza-e-tabiee). These organs are identified as:

(a) Nutritive Organs, and

(b) Genital Organs.

(a) nutritive organs are of two types:

- The digestive organs include:

- oral cavity

- teeth
- salivary glands
- pharynx
- esophagus
- stomach
- Intestine
- liver
- gall bladder
- pancreas
- spleen
- other endocrine glands

▪ Excretory Organs include:

- Kidneys
- Ureters
- Urinary bladder
- Urethra (Urethra)

(b) Genital Organs:

▪ Male Genital Organs:

- Testes

- Epididymis
- Vas deferens
- Seminal vesicles
- Ejaculatory Duct
- Penis
- Prostrate
- Bulbo-urethral glands

▪ Female Genital Organs:

- Ovary
- Uterus
- Uterine Tube
- Vagina
- Vulva

II: Psychic/Mental Organs (aza-e-nafsani)

Compound organs pertaining to ghova-e-nafsani and afaal-e-nafsani are known as aza-e-nafsani. These organs are concerned with the perception of sensory stimuli, their conduction, integration, retention and conversion into motor signals, and conduction to the effector organs for final motor function. The functions of conceiving or thought, intelligence, and cognition are also concerned with these organs.

Psychic/mental organs are classified into:

- **Central Organs:**

- Brain
- Fore Brain
- Mid Brain
- Hind Brain
- Spinal Cord

- **Peripheral Organs:**

- Cranial Nerves
- Spinal Nerves
- Nerve Ganglia
- Eye, Ear, Nose
- Tongue
- Skin
- Muscles acting under the motor faculty

III: The Vital Organs (aza-e-hayati)

Compound in structure, these are the organs pertaining to circulation of blood and respiration:

- Heart
- Arteries
- Veins

- Capillaries
- Larynx
- Trachea
- Bronchi
- Bronchioles
- Lungs
- Thorax
- Pleurae
- Diaphragm

IV: The Essential Organs (aza-e-raeese)

The number of vital organs is same as there are *necessary faculties* in the body. And since there are three necessary faculties for the preservation of "individual" and one for the preservation of "species", therefore according to the preservation and succession phenomenon, Essential Organs are identified as four in number:

Heart

Brain

Liver

Testes and Ovaries

▪ **Heart:** It serves vital force (ghovat-e-hayavani) and supplies nutrition and pneumatic support to all organs and thereby their vitality is ensured. Heart is considered the center of vital force.

- **Brain:**

According to psychic faculty (ghovat-e-nafsani) it is one of the essential organs. Serving psychic faculty, it is responsible for all sensations and movements in the body. Brain is considered as the center of all psychic/mental faculties.

- **Liver:**

According to natural faculty (ghovat-e-tabiee), it is the essential organ serves the natural faculty, especially the nutritive faculties, and is responsible for nearly all metabolic functions in the body. Liver is considered the center of whole nutritive faculties.

- **Testes and Ovaries:**

According to the faculties of reproduction, these are the essential organs, responsible for preservation and propagation of species, considered as the centers of reproductive faculties.

These (four) essential organs are assumed practically to be self-sufficient and self-sustaining with respect to their own faculties. But for other power faculties they have to depend on other vital organs. As for example the brain which is self- sufficient in psychic faculty which is its personal and real faculty, but it has to depend for vital & natural faculty on the heart and liver respectively. Similarly, heart is furnished with vital faculty which is, the real and self-power of the heart but it depends for the sensations and movements on the brain and for correct physiological functions on the liver.

The Vital Force (pneuma/ spirit)

There are certain faculties or the powers and 'drives' of the body corresponding to the three biological systems physical, nervous and vital. Physical faculty is responsible for nutrition and growth and is centered in the liver. The nervous faculty provides sensation and movement and is centered in the brain. The vital faculty is a prerequisite to life and activity of every organ and tissue. The vital faculty expands and contracts the vital force and moves it inwards and outwards. It brings in light and air to condition the vital force and expels the hot smoky vapors for its purification. Hence, from the point of view of life, the vital faculty imparts reactivity to the vital force and from the point of pulse and respiration, it endows it with activity.

Due to the confusion of the term with 'soul' it has been associated with 'nafs' or i.e. something personal to each individual, immaterial and immortal, Somtimes refers to a physical body (organism) endowed with a self-directing purposeful energy. Galen deemed 'rooh' as the breath (Pneuma).

But Avicenna holds that vital force is not what the philosophers call the 'soul or anima', it is a luminous substance, a ray of light which emerges from a mixture of the first principles, and approaches towards likeness of the celestial beings. Later on it has been resolved according to the principles of Persian Medicine that 'it is a subtle vapor which rises from the blood, diffuses itself to the remotest arteries, and resembles the sun in luminosity'.

As a luminous substance the celestial vital force is formed of the light vapors portions of Humors, it is carried by the heart and blood vessels, is purified by the inspiration of light air [0_2] and is moderated by the expiration of hot smoky vapor [$C0_2$& H_20]. The vital force as a substance may, therefore, be identified with the immediately combustible moiety of the nutriment [and thus with the glucose and its auxiliaries such as the hormones, vitamins and enzymes].

As a ray of light vital force is the "innate heat" or vital energy, which is 'the instrument of all the faculties' and which moves with the vital force. During sleep the vital force moves inwards the innate heat too moves with it and thus strengthens the physical faculty but leaves the exterior of the body cold, and so the nervous faculty dull and sluggish. The opposite happens in the case of wakefulness. Similarly, when in fear the vital force moves inwards the exterior becomes cold and the interior hot. In anger the opposite occurs the outer nervous faculty becomes activated while the inner physical one is dulled.

The vital faculty which thus supplies energy maintains the body temperature, heart beats and respiratory movements are identifiable with the basal metabolism of the body.

The centers of the autonomic nervous system in the brain and spinal cord which control the quantitative discharge of the vital force through contraction and expansion of the pulse, direct its qualitative discharge by inward [anabolic] and outward [catabolic] movement of vital energy through the sympathetic and Para-sympathetic routes such as during sleep and wakefulness, and in emotions of fear and anger, may be recognized as center or 'heart' of the vital faculty.

According to Avicenna 'The foundation or beginning of all these faculties is traceable to the heart, as is agreed upon even by those philosophers who think that the source of visual, auditory and gustatory power lies in the brain". This 'heart', however, is not just the structural heart described by the anatomists but the functional heart which as the center of emotions, thermo-regulation, sleep and water metabolism is centered in the diencephalon, a portion of the brain which in the phylogeny of race was the first to develop. The pituitary which sub serves as well as regulates the functions of this region may also be included in the concept of the 'heart' described in the Canon.

This generalization of the various organs and systems under the heading of faculties and vital forces lacks the wealth of detail available in modern physiology but it offers the picture of man as a Psychosomatic unity of interacting physical, nervous and emotional factors and provides a better understanding of the dual aspects of the heart - one of circulation and other of emotions'.

Source of Vital Force

It has been established by almost all the physicians that *rooh* in fact is a gaseous substance whose source is the atmospheric air when the inspired air reaches the alveoli of the lungs; the oxygen part of air is absorbed by blood, becomes the part of the body and thus called 'rooh'. Oxygen outside the body is not called *'rooh'* but it is a simple (elementary) constituent of atmospheric air.

However, when it is absorbed in the red blood corpuscles and fluids &humors of the body it becomes so (for the body). Galen identified blood as carrier of vital force. This rooh-e-hayavani enters the lungs from the air through respiration and then reaches to the heart and becomes the source of production of heat (energy). It has also been mentioned by Persian Medicine Physicians that the source of *rooh* is air which is inhaled through respiration.

Avicenna states that this air is not only an *element* for our bodies and vital forces but it is a help which continuously reaches in our body and becomes the cause of its promotion, not only in the capacity of being element but for being an active agent too.

Persian Medicine holds that there is no organ in the body left without *rooh*. Where there is blood, there is *rooh*. Tissue fluid also contains rooh. The organs which are not supplied with blood, their supply of *rooh* are met with or by other humors (fluids), which carry it to those structures. However, it is said that arterial blood contains more *rooh* than the venous, but the pulmonary arteries contain less *rooh* than the pulmonary veins. Similarly, left chambers of the heart contain more *rooh* than the right chambers. Similarly, the organs whose temperament is hot, are more active and their metabolic rate is very high, contain more *rooh*; contrary to this, the organs whose temperament is cold contain less *rooh*. Thus, the consumption of it in an organ clearly indicates the temperament of that organ with respect to its hotness or coldness.

Functions of *rooh* (pneuma)

The physicians have enumerated the following functions which are virtually the results of the same process:

- Pneuma produces innate or real or normal heat (hararat-e-gharizi) in the body.

- Pneumaproduces energy in the body which keeps all the faculties functioning.

- Pneumakeeps all the organs of the body alive.

Production of Energy and Heat by the pneuma

It is well known to us that a process of metabolic changes is going on in our body. This metabolism (estehaleh) is composed of two processes: (1) anabolism and (2) catabolism. With the result of these *metabolisms* production of energy in the form of ATP and heat, takes place. In this production of energy and heat two important factors from *omoor-e-tabieeye* of our body participate:

- Pneuma, which is obtained from the inspired air.

- Fine humors (nutrients), which are obtained from the blood plasma.

When action and reaction among pneuma and fine humors takes place, or in other words burning (ehteragh) of nutriments takes place with the pneuma, the energy and heat are produced, thereby the organs of the body become able to continue their respective functions. It is why Abu Sahl Masihi has called the *nutrients* as *fuel* and the external air as *precursor of pneuma.*

The example of the internal burning in the microcosm (human body) is given by the physicians with the burning of coal or glowing of lamp in the outside world (macrocosm). They maintain that as the heat is produced by the burning of coal or the lamp, in the same manner there is a fuel, like coal or oil in the body which when meets the pneuma, gets burnt.

The only difference between the two oxidation (ehteragh) is that the process of production of energy and heat is organized-one in the body and the energy is released in an organized and controlled manner, whereas in the external world the coal is burnt abruptly and the energy is also released abruptly. The internal heat is released with normalcy (etedal) which is essential for the maintenance of health. This very normal heat is called as innate heat.

When the heat exceeds the normal limits, it is called fever or hyperpyrexia (homma, hararat-e-gharibeh), or when it falls below normal it is called as hypopyrexia.

With the result of this oxidation waste product of pneuma are produced (fazleh-e-rooh, bokharat-e-dokhani) which is now known as carbon dioxide. Excretion of these wastes from the body is essential. While discussing the functions of respiration Avicenna has clearly mentioned two functions:

Oxygenation (tarvih): i.e. furnishing of pneumato the organs.

Excretion (tanghiyeh): i.e. expelling of *bokharat-e-dokhani* ($C0_2$) from the body.

Faculties and pneuma

The Persian Medicine holds that the maintenance and proper functioning of faculties depends upon the continuous supply of pneuma. Any cessation of the supply of pneuma means cessation in the functioning of faculties. It has already been seen that when with the help of pneuma, fine humors (glucose, amino acids, fatty acids and glycerol) undergo oxidation, huge amount of energy in the form of adenosine triphosphate (ATP) and heat is produced. This very energy (ATP) causes to perform the chemical, physical and mechanical functions in the body. Thus, this energy is a constant source of supply to all faculties. In other words, the faculties of the body will continue their functioning as long as the general energy (ATP) remains available to the respective organs which are center of these faculties. That is why it is generally held that all the bodily faculties exist owing to the dynamics of pneuma.

Kinds of pneuma

In accordance with three faculties, pneuma has also been divided into three kinds: natural pneuma, vital pneuma and psychic pneuma. When the pneum are aches to the liver the center of natural faculty, it is called as natural pneuma, where it produces general energy to help natural faculty. Similarly, when it reaches to the heart the center of vital faculty, it is called as vital pneuma, where it helps vital faculty to discharge its functions; and likewise when the pneuma reaches to the brain the center of psychic faculty, it is called as psychic pneuma, where it helps psychic faculty to perform its functions. Thus, the essence of pneuma is the same, but the difference is only of the names. The name of the pneuma varies according to respective vital organs particularly for each of the faculties.

A fact should also be borne in mind that in between pneuma and faculties there is an intermediary thing and that is general energy in the form of ATP. And though this general energy is produced in each and every cell of the body, but in vital organs it performs specialized functions by potentiating the respective faculties which perform specialized functions pertaining to their respective faculties. Therefore, that general energy which is produced by that particular pneuma which reaches the vital organs is called as natural pneuma, vital pneuma and psychic pneuma.

Somtimes the meanings of natural pneuma, vital pneuma and psychic pneuma are taken as natural faculty, vital faculty and psychic faculty. Here also these terms signify the presence of some types of energy in between pneuma and faculties, which plays paramount role in the functioning of faculties.

Faculties

The faculties are those natural and specialized powers which are furnished to a living body for the performance of its special functions, and which become cause for the performance of the body, for the preservation of the individual as well as species. No organ is devoid of this power or Functional Faculty. There are three major divisions of Faculties/ Functional Power of the body:

Kinds of faculties:

- Natural Faculties.

- Physical or Mental Faculties.

▪ Vital Faculties.

The concept of Faculties/Powers is unique in Persian Medicine. The Faculty is that property of the body with which the phenomenon of life is manifested. Faculty provides the basis for different body functions as described in the following discussion.

Natural Faculty

Natural faculties are those which are responsible for ingestion of Food and excretion of waste products; and preservation of race. The organs pertaining to this faculty are called *natural organs*. The chief organ or the seat or center of this faculty is the liver.

Kinds of Natural Faculty

According to the above function, natural faculties have been divided into the following three faculties:

▪ Nutritive Faculty.

▪ The Faculty of Growth (ghova-e-naamiye).

▪ Reproductive Faculty (ghova-e-tanasoli).

Kinds of Nutritive Faculty

According to the above functions the above faculty has been divided into the following Faculty (Powers):

1. Power of Attraction or Ingestion (jazebeh).

2. Retentive Power (masekeh).

3. Power of Digestion or Transformation (hazameh, moghayer-e-sani)

4. Power of Propulsion or Excretion (dafe-e).

According to Persian Medicine each of the above four Faculties are two-fold:

- One is that which attract the external food and sends it to the stomach (gastro-intestinal tract) then retains it and transforms into the materials capable of becoming the blood and then transfer it towards the liver. All these changes do not take place in the lumen of the latter (this transformation is called simple digestion in the gastro-intestinal tract).

- The other one is that which is found in the substance (Cells) of the gastro-intestinal tract and attracts the Food into the cells, then retains it there and transforms it into the likeness of substance of the gastrointestinal tract and expels the Waste Products. The same thing also takes place in the liver. This is organ digestion (hazm-e-ozvi).

Therefore, the above four Faculty (Powers) are twofold, one found in the gastro-intestinal tract to complete the whole process of digestion (Ingestion, Retention, Digestion and Expulsion) and the same are found in all the cells of the body which absorb the food materials, pneuma, metabolize and transform them into various compounds and replace the wear and tear and produce the Faculty (Energy) for the proper functioning of different Faculties.

Reproductive Faculties

Reproductive Faculties are other kinds of Natural Faculties which act on the Food for the preservation of species. These faculties ensure propagation and preservation of the species to replace what is lost through the death of its members. These faculties are responsible for the generation of Semen i.e. *sperm and ovum*; for all sexual functions and formation of the fetus in the mother's womb.

These faculties are of two kinds.

- Generative Faculty (ghova-e-movalledeh).

- Formative Faculty (ghova-e-mosavereh).

Generative Faculty:

According to Persian Medicine this is the Faculty which separates the essence of semen i.e. sperm or ovum, from compounds of the body inside the testis (and Ovary) and makes each of its part to become a particular organ.

Avicenna is of the opinion that ***Generative Faculty*** is of two kinds: one kind generates sperm and ovum in the males and females respectively, and the other one is that which gives different combination to different potentialities of the sperm and ovum, according to future organs. This Faculty is also called Primary Transformative Power (ghova-e-movalehe-e-ulla).

Formative Faculty

According to Persian Medicine the other faculty gives shape to each part of sperm and ovum which is required by that particular species to which this sperm and ovum belongs, or any other shape close to that particular individual. Giving of shape means it produces lines in the organs, forms cavities and depressions and performs other functions. This Faculty is known as *formative faculty*. Avicenna says the formative faculty is that whereby, subject to the decree of Allah, delineation and configuration of the organs is produced with all their cavities, foramina, positions and relations to one another, their smoothness or roughness and so on - all being controlled up to the final limits of their natural dimension. ***Ali ibn abbas*** had also of the same opinion.

This Faculty controls the following functions:

- Male and Female sexual powers (potency) and functions of copulation.
- Fertilization of ovum.
- Transplantation of ovum.
- Cleavage and differentiation of ovum.

- Formation of membranes and fetal parts.

- Development of ovum (Fetus).

- Parturition.

- Psychic or Mental Faculties

These are those faculties which perform intellectual, sensory and motor functions in the body. In the other words they perform all the functions of the nervous system. The organs pertaining to these are brain, spinal cord and nerves etc. And the brain itself is considered to be the supreme member of this group i.e. the seat of psychic faculty.

This major faculty is composed of three faculties.

- Perceptive faculties (ghova-e-hasaseh, modrekeh).

- motor faculties(ghova-e-moharekeh)

- faculty of planning and mind or intellectual faculties

(Ghova-e-modabbereh)

- Internal perceptive faculties (This is called by Avicenna and his followers as ghova-e-modrekeh-e-baateni.

Faculties of Perception

Perceptive Faculties receive all kinds of sensory stimuli from different sensory receptors and send it to the brain in their respective internal centers. These are of two kinds.

- External Perceptive Faculties

(Ghova-e-moderekeh-e-zaheri)

- Internal Perceptive Faculties

(Ghova-e-modrekeh-e-baateni).

External Perceptive Faculties

These sensory faculties are composed of five faculties related to five external sense organs.

- *Power of Vision* related to the Eyes.

- *Power of Hearing* related to the Ears.

- *Power of Smell* related to the Nose.

- *Power of Taste* related to the Tongue.

- *Power of Tactile Sensations* related to the Skin etc.

Internal Perceptive Faculties

These are internal perceptive faculties which recognize and perceive the particular forms and meanings of those particular things that have been perceived by the external senses. The number of these internal perceptive faculties is five according to five external perceptive stimuli. The followings are these faculties with their centers in the brain.

- Internal Visual Faculty

Its center is the occipital lobe of the cerebrum especially the calcarine sulcus. In area 17 the visual impulses are received and the form of the object is perceived (visual sensory area). In area 18 the exact meaning of a visual image is interpreted and integrated such as the meaning of written language (visual psychic area).

- Internal Hearing Faculty

The center of this faculty is temporal lobe of the cerebrum. In area 41, 42 (Herschel's Gyrus) and adjoining part of Superior temporal gyrus (Area 22) the pitch, loudness and quality (form) of the sound are perceived. The center is bilateral.

▪ Internal Faculty of Smell

Its center is situated in the uncus and hippocampal gyrus (cerebrum). Here olfactory sensations are perceived.

▪ Internal Gustatory Faculty

Its center is situated in the inferior part of the post central gyrus in cerebrum. Here general sensation and sensation of taste is perceived.

▪ Internal Faculty for General Sensation

The centers for perception of touch, temperature (heat, cold), pain, kinesthetic sensations are situated in somesthetic area parietal lobe of cerebrum. Area 3, 2, 1 are the perception areas for perceiving the form of the general sensations and areas 5, 7 are the psychic association area for perceiving the meaning.

Thus, the complete meaning of the particular sensation is understood such as:

a) Appreciation of the size, shape, texture and weight of the object Steriognosis;

b) Appreciation of the relative intensity of different stimuli; c) tactile localization, tactile discrimination of two points, recognition of position and passive movements of the limbs.

According to Avicenna who accepted the views of ancient

Philosophers instead of the physicians, the five internal

Perceptive or sensory faculties are:

▪ Faculty of Common sense (hes-e-moshtarak)

- Faculty of Imagination (a type of memory) (khial)

- Faculty of Apprehension (vahm).

- Faculty of Ideation (motekhayele, mofakereh, motesavereh)

- Faculty of retention (hafezeh).

Motor Faculties

Almost all sensory and even the abstract experiences of the mind are eventually expressed in some type of motor activity, such as actual muscular movements of direct nature, contraction or relaxation of the muscles, attainment of posture, crying and laughing etc. Thus Motor Faculty is that power which becomes cause for all the bodily movements.

Motor Faculty controls the motor activities in the following sequence of three stages.

- First the thought is originated for the motor activity to be performed. Thereafter,

- The sequence of movements necessary to perform the overall task is determined. And lastly,

- The muscular movements themselves are controlled.

Thus, according to these stages, Persian Medicine has classified this Faculty (Power) into following four kinds.

- Power of Ideation or Thinking (ghova-e-khial, vahm)

- Desiring Faculty (ghova-e-shoghiyeh)

- Faculty of Determination (ghova-e-tamiz)

- Efficient or Operational Faculty (ghova-e-feliyeh)

Intellectual Faculties

These faculties are called as Faculty of Planning (tadbir) or Mind (zehn) and Thought (fekr) classified into three categories:

- Takhayyol or motekhayyeleh
- Fekr or mofakkereh
- Zekr or motezakereh

Avicenna and his associates, who have followed the views of philosophers instead of the physicians, have called this faculty as Internal Perceptive Faculties and have classified these into the five categories as under:

1. Faculty of Commonsense
2. Faculty of Imagination (a type of memory)
3. Faculty of Apprehension
4. Faculty of Ideation
5. Faculty of retention

Thought, Memory, Learning and Consciousness are all the function of the intellectual faculty of the brain.

Vital Faculties

Vital Faculties are those faculties which furnish vitality to the organs enable them to receive Mental Power to accomplish various activities of life. The organs concerned with this faculty are known as vital organs.

"Vital faculty has been defined as those faculties due to which the life is maintained, and whose seat is the heart. These begin from the heart, enter the arteries and reach all over the body and furnish life to them. Among these Faculties One Faculty (Power) is *Efficient Power* which causes contraction and relaxation in the heart and arteries".

In fact, vital faculty is the faculty which is the source of life for the organs. Thus life is maintained by the following two processes:

- By the process of respiration —whereby the air is inspired and pneuma is absorbed by the lungs from the inspired air and Waste Product of pneum i.e. Carbon dioxide) is exhaled from the lungs.

- By the process of blood circulation —whereby the blood circulates all over the body with the pumping action of the heart, thus pneuma is absorbed by the blood in the lungs and carried to the heart, which pumps the pneuma and fine humors (Nutriments to all cells and tissues) to be metabolized by natural faculty to produce general energy (vital pnema, natural pneuma, and psychic pneuma) to serve various Faculty (Faculties) of the body to carry on various activities of life. Carbon dioxide produced with the result of *oxidation* of finc humors (Nutriments), are carried to the lungs with the venous blood, to be expelled out by the process of expiration.

Functions

Since Functions and Faculties are inseparable and these are functions that are tesPersian Medicineony to the presence of Faculty, therefore, Functions are as many as there are Faculties. Functions have already been described with the discussion of the Faculties. However, it is customary to give a general description of functions under a separate heading.

Classification of Functions

- According to Faculty (Faculties)

- According to the number of Faculty (Powers) subservient to particular function.

Classification of Functions According to Faculties

- **Natural Functions**
  - Function of Nutrition
  - Function of Growth
  - Function of Reproduction

These functions have been further subdivided into different functions according to further subdivision of different Natural Faculties.

- **Mental or Psychic Functions**
  - Sensory Function
  - Motor Function
  - Intellectual Function.

These functions have been again subdivided into different functions, according to further subdivision of different psychic Faculty.

- **Vital Functions**
  - Blood Circulation
  - Respiration

These functions have been further subdivided into various other functions.

Classification of functions according to number of Faculty (Power) participating in a function.

- simple function

▪ compound function

▪ **Simple functions:** Simple functions are those which are carried out by single faculty (power) under any of the faculties.

o Example under natural faculty

a. Attraction or absorption (jazebeh) which is performed by simple diffusion or active transport. Pinocytosis also belongs to this category. Physicians have described three physical forces i.e. magnet like attraction, suction like roots of the trees, and vacuum like action.

b. Retention (masekeh) of material inside the cells.

c. Function of transformation (hazm), anabolism and catabolism inside the cells also belong to the category of simple functions.

d. Function of expulsion (dafe-e) waste products and other materials not needed to the cell are expelled out. Functions of attraction (tahsil), adhesion (elzagh) and assimilation (tashbih) also belong to simple functions (afaal-e-mofrad).

o Examples under psychic faculty: Depolarization, development of action potential and conduction of impulse through the neurons and contraction of the muscle fibers.

o Examples under vital faculty: Exchange of gases (rooh and dokhan) in the lungs and tissues and production of general energy in the form of ATP or vital pneuma. However, the exchange of gases takes place under natural faculty.

▪ **Compound functions (afaal-e-morakab)** compound functions are those which are performed by more than one power.

o Examples under natural faculty

a. Mastication of food

b. Deglutition

c. Digestion of food in gastro-intestinal tract

d. Propulsion and defecation

e. Formation of urine etc.

- **Examples under psychic faculty**

a. Foundation of sight, hearing, smell, taste, and tactile sensations.

b. Various voluntary and involuntary movements, e.g. speech, locomotion, and movements of visceral muscles.

c. Function of thought, ideation, memory and other

d. Intellectual functions.

- **Examples under vital faculty**

a. Respiration

b. Systole and diastole of the heart, whereby blood circulation is achieved.

c. Vasoconstriction and dilatation action under psychic faculty

Although the above functions have been classified under each of three faculties but many of these functions are combined actions of more than one faculty i.e. inter-faculty actions.

The Six Essential Principles

The Origins of Health and Disease

Hygiene is the art of personal health maintenance and disease prevention. Persian Medicine is, at its core, basically just an elaborate and sophisticated system of hygiene.

In proper hygiene practices, Persian Medicine sees the foundation of all good health. In improper or faulty hygiene, Persian Medicine sees the origin of most disease.

The art of hygiene is basically twofold, like the two sides of a coin. On the one side, you must give your body all the good things it needs: a pure, wholesome, nutritious diet; appropriate and adequate physical activity and exercise; sufficient sleep and rest; and a healthy, constructive daily routine and lifestyle. On the other hand, you must remove from the body all the wastes and pathogenic matter that it doesn't need, by keeping it clean, both inside and out.

Persian Medicine has identified six basic areas or factors which, if kept in good order, build health and which, if allowed to fall into disorder, lead to illness and disease. They constitute the basis of all health management and disease prevention in Persian Medicine, and are as follows:

1) Ambient Air

2) Food and Drink

3) Exercise and Rest

4) Sleep and Wakefulness

5) Retention and Evacuation of Wastes

6) Perturbations of the Mind and Emotions

Because these six factors are not essentially inherent to the body and its nature, they are Somtimes called the Six Non-Natural Factors. Because they concern important aspects of hygiene, I call them the Six Hygienic Factors.

The proper management of these six factors constitutes the entire art of hygiene in Persian Medicine. To recapitulate on the Six Essential Principles and what they entail:

Ambient Air: The impact of one's habitat and dwelling place on one's health: The influence of geographic, seasonal, climactic and environmental factors on one's health, The art of proper breathing, The basis of all public health and environmental medicine. (51)

Food and Drink: The basics of a healthy diet, proper food selection and healthy eating habits. Constitutional management with diet: Not just what you eat, but also when, where, how and how much.

Exercise and Rest: The value and importance of proper exercise, the different types of exercise, and selecting the right one, how to design a safe, effective, sensible and appropriate exercise routine and regimen, Finding the right balance between exercise and rest.

Sleep and Wakefulness: The importance and value of adequate sleep in health maintenance, designing a healthful daily routine that balances adequate, sound, restful sleep with appropriate, constructive wakeful activity. Harmonizing one's personal sleep / wake cycles with the rhythms of Nature.

Retention and Evacuation of Wastes: Recognizing and cultivating the right balance between waste retention and waste evacuation, building healthy bowel habits, maintaining urinary health. Recognizing, preventing and treating autointoxication, Simple hygienic cleansing measures.

Perturbations of the Mind and Emotions: The impact of our mental and emotional states on our health, Constitutional management of the mind and emotions, Appropriate, satisfying, affectionate and constructive sexual relations.

Ambient air

Environmental Medicine

The human organism can live for a few days without water, and for several days without food. But deny it air and its life-giving pneuma, and the body will die within minutes.

Because the air we breathe is so vitally and immediately important to the health of the entire organism, Ambient Air is the first of the Six Essential Principles to consider. Air and its pneuma are the essential food for the Vital Faculty, which gives life to the whole organism. Because the Vital Faculty supports and underlies the health and functioning of the entire organism, our overall health and vitality can only be as good as the quality and quantity of the air we breathe.

The air we breathe is all around us. And so, the essential factor of Ambient Air includes many other factors and considerations - climactic, seasonal, geographic and environmental. It forms the basis of classical Iranian environmental medicine and public health.

Because the air we breathe is free and invisible, it's so often taken for granted. But the discerning physician, in assessing the patient's health, will always inquire about his/her living environment and the air he/she breathes.

Dwelling Place and Living Environment

The site or location of one's house or dwelling is an important factor in considerations of ambient air. Above all, balance and the Golden Mean between extremes are desired.

The home or dwelling should be well ventilated and not stuffy, but neither should it be exposed to wind, drafts, or chills. It shouldn't be on a high, windy ridge, but neither should it be totally enclosed or surrounded by high walls that shut out all light and fresh air.

The ideal dwelling place should receive a moderate amount of sunlight, not too glaring or direct, and tempered by an adequate amount of refreshing shade for contrast. There should be sufficient light and not too much shadow and gloom.

The temperature of one's dwelling should be moderate. There should be adequate heating and hot during the winter months, and protection from cold drafts and chills. In the summer, it shouldn't be too hot, and should be exposed to fresh, cool breezes.

The ancient Iranians realized that the stale, foul air around swamps breeds disease, so they had swamps drained, especially around major cities and population centers. Above all, one's home or dwelling should be free from foul, noxious odors and vapors.

Climate and Country

The Iranian physician always considers or makes concessions for the patient's country and its prevailing climactic conditions in assessing the patient's health. If possible, adjustments should be made to compensate for extremes in climate.

The ancient Iranians considered themselves to be blessed to live in a country with a temperate, sunny climate that wasn't too hot in the summer or too cold in the winter. They recognized that extremes of heat, cold, moisture or dryness placed added stresses and burdens on the individual and his/her health.

Environments that are extremely hot and sunny also tend to be excessively dry; such are arrid desert environments. Over the long term, they tend to wither, dry and emaciate the individual. However, they may be therapeutic or remedial for those suffering from cold, wet afflictions like chronic bronchitis, weeping eczema, or rheumatism.

Environments that are hot and humid, often in tropical climates, tend to be heavy and oppressive, and the air hard to breathe. They tend to breed infectious diseases. Otherwise, they are not particularly conducive to energy and vitality. Proper cleanliness and hygiene are imperative in such climes and seasons.

Environments that are cold, dark and moist tend to be depressing, and will aggravate chronic Phlegmatic conditions like rheumatism, bronchitis and asthma. The excessive cold and dampness puts a great strain on the immune system to protect against colds and flu.

Environments that are cold and dry aggravate Melancholic conditions like dry skin, arthritis, rheumatism, and nervous, spasmodic afflictions. Often, these are high altitude mountainous or high desert environments, which are also frequently plagued by strong winds, which also aggravate nervous, spasmodic afflictions. Since the evaporation rate is higher in high altitude environments, proper and adequate hydration is extremely important.

Persian Medicine also recognizes the beneficial effect that the air of mountainous environments, as well as seaside environments, has upon the health. In particular, such airs tend to promote good digestion and good sleep.

Seasonal Influences on Health

The physiology and functioning of the human organism cannot remain constant, but must adapt to seasonal changes and variations in the weather. An important part of being healthy is having the necessary flexibility and adaptability to adjust to seasonal changes in the weather.

The response of the organism to seasonal weather changes is coordinated by the Vital Faculty through the respiratory, circulatory and immune systems. However, the humors and the

Natural Faculty, as well as the other faculties and systems of the organism, are also affected.

In winter, the cold, wet weather aggravates phlegm, and makes us vulnerable to coughs, colds and lung congestion. Since our bodies consume more energy to keep us Hot, our caloric needs are higher in winter. And so, we must eat a heavier, richer, heartier diet. The cold weather also shunts the majority of the blood circulation into the interior to hot the vital organs of the body's core. Similarly, humoral superfluities and imbalances are driven deep into the body's interior, and remain latent during the winter. The colder winter temperatures make the maturation and ripening of the humors slower, and humoral disorders take longer to manifest.

In spring, the Hoter weather brings the formerly latent or dormant humoral excesses of winter up to the surface. The excessive phlegm accumulated during the winter months starts to resurface to be passed off. This surfacing of phlegm can aggravate or manifest spring pollen allergies and hay fever. Because all the accumulated excesses and superfluities of winter are being passed off, spring is a good season for fasting and cleansing regimes, which shouldn't be undertaken until the last cold snaps of winter are over. Blood also gets more exuberant and rises to the surface, making bleeding disorders like nosebleeds a problem in the spring. Wind is also strong and abundant in the spring, so one must take care to protect oneself against drafts and chills.

In summer, the hot weather shunts blood out to the exterior of the organism and the superficial capillaries in order to disperse excess heat from the body's interior. If more cooling and heat dispersal are needed, the body breaks a sweat. The hot, dry summer weather provokes aggravations of heat and choler, or yellow bile. These may produce giddiness, vomiting or nausea, as well as fevers, infections, putrefactions, heat rashes and inflammatory conditions. Because more blood is shunted out towards the exterior of the organism, the digestive organs in the body's core don't receive as much blood. This, plus the lower caloric needs of summer, often tends to depress the appetite; in summer, we should eat light, easy to digest foods. Also, since the intense summer heat leads to a lot of fluid loss through sweating, we must drink a lot of fluids to keep ourselves well-hydrated. Since the humors ripen more quickly in hot weather, humoral diseases are more active in summer, and run their course in a shorter period of time.

As summer moves into fall, the days remain hot, but the nights grow colder. These widening temperature fluctuations put a strain on the organism to adapt. The pores may open and sweat during the heat of the day, and allow evening chills to enter. Excess cold foods and drinks consumed in summer may have generated superfluous cold, damp Phlegmatic humors that may increase one's vulnerability to chills when the weather starts changing in the fall. One should take care not to drink too many cold drinks nor eat too many cooling foods when the weather starts changing. The cold, dry weather of mid-fall can produce dry, chapped skin, coryza and sore throats, coughs and hoarseness, and can aggravate Melancholic complaints. Wetter autumns are better than dryer ones, because the moisture in the air will help to liquefy the excess phlegm accumulated through dietary indiscretions in the summer, whereas dryness will only dry up and thicken this excess phlegm, making it more difficult to expel.

As the weather becomes colder again towards winter, the caloric needs of the organism increase, and the diet becomes heavier. Cold, wet winter weather produces coughs, colds and lung congestion, and the blood circulation starts to interiorize to hot the body's core. The wheel of the seasons has again come full circle.

Diet: food and drink

How to Eat for Optimum Health

After the air we breathe, the next in importance is diet, or the influence of food and drink on health. A pure, natural, wholesome nutritious diet is essential to good health.

Because most of the substances we take into our bodies are items of food and drink consumed in our daily diet, what we eat and drink has an enormous impact on our health. And, unlike the ambient air, we exercise much more control over what we eat.

And so, diet and dietary therapy are the main modalities or tools of health management and disease prevention in Persian Medicine. The great advantages of working with diet are that foods are safe, gentle and effective, and have a very low level of toxicity.

Because the natural herbal medicines and remedies used in Persian Medicine are usually gentler and milder than modern pharmaceutical drugs, the diet consumed during treatment must support and be congruent with the direction and aim of the therapy. Ulimately, the success of natural herbal medicines and therapy is greatly reduced, or even nullified altogether if not accompanied by the right diet.

Pure Water

The most important and most frequently consumed drink is water. The water drunk must be clear, pure and free of microbes, pollutants and impurities. Its taste should be mild and sweet, and it should be soft, and free from any hard, harsh mineral residues. Fresh mountain spring water is the best. Securing a good source of pure, fresh water is the first and most basic foundation of a good, healthy diet.

The water drunk should be moderately cool or at room temperature, but not ice cold. Ice cold drinks are unnatural, and compromise the circulation, immunity and digestive power of the organism with cold, wet Phlegmatic humors.

The Basics of a Natural Diet

When we select and prepare the foods in our diet, we should take care to consume them in as natural a state as possible. The more we process, refine, or alter the food from its natural state, the more we compromise its inherent vitality, wholeness and nutritional value.

All refined sugars, starches and carbohydrates should be avoided wherever possible. In their place should be put whole grains and natural sweeteners.

Foods that have not been artificially processed, or that have been minimally processed, should take precedence over those that have been highly or unnaturally processed. All hydrogenated fats should be eliminated.

Food additives and preservatives should also be greatly reduced or eliminated. Some preservatives are more natural than others, whereas some are toxic and dangerous. Most linger as a residue in the organism, impeding its vitality and functioning.

The Nature and Temperament of Foods

Persian Medicine assesses the nature and temperament of foods, and their impact on the organism, primarily in terms of the Four Basic Qualities: Hot, Cold, Wet and Dry. This enables us to personalize our food selection, giving preference to foods that complement or remedy imbalances, either innate or acquired, of humor and temperament.

Since Hot / Cold are the primary or active polarity, our first consideration must be to the heating or cooling nature of foods. Heating foods are those which stimulation the metabolism, whereas cooling foods are those which sedate the metabolism and relieve excess heat. Examples are as follows:

Hot: garlic, onions, horseradish, ginger, chicken, eggs, duck, lamb, wheat, sesame seeds, walnuts, apples, olives and aged cheeses.

Cold: milk and dairy products, fresh cheeses, yogurt, most tropical fruits, lettuce, cucumber, watermelon, fish.

Dry / Wet is the passive or secondary polarity. Wet foods are those which are unctuous, rich, oily, moistening and emollient. Dry foods are those which are either physically dry, or those which aid the organism in eliminating excess fluids. Examples are:

Dry: most beans, soybeans, pomegranates, asparagus, dried fruits, aged cheeses.

Wet: milk and dairy products, bananas, avocados, coconut, fresh cheeses, yogurt.

Closely related to the Dry / Wet polarity are the qualities of Light and Heavy, respectively. Light foods produce lightness, alertness and agility in the body, but in excess, they can lead to lightheadedness, spiciness and emaciation. Heavy foods, of high quality, can give strength and durability to the body, but most commonly they produce sluggishness, heaviness and drowsiness, and are difficult to digest.

Light: rice cakes, popcorn, corn, sunflower seeds

Heavy: beef, wheat, eggplant, greasy fried foods.

I don't want to get excessively hairsplitting or dogmatic here, but I do want to cultivate in you an awareness and sensitivity to the effects of the foods we eat upon our health.

Foods and the Four Humors

Each one of the Four Humors has certain foods that aggravate it. Consumption of these foods should be greatly reduced or avoided by those with an excess or aggravation of that humor, whether it be innate and constitutional, or an acquired condition or imbalance. The main problematic or aggravating foods for each humor are:

Phlegm: milk, dairy products, fresh cheeses, refined sugar, refined starches and flours, wheat and glutinous foods, cold foods, ice cold drinks; moist, creamy rich foods.

Yellow Bile: salt and salty foods, fats and cholesterol, fried foods, vinegar, alcohol, excessive sour or fermented foods, aged cheeses, excessive hot spices and chilies, excessive beef and red meat.

Black Bile: old, dry stale foods: excessive beans, soy, nuts, astringent foods, peanuts, rancid fats, nightshade vegetables - especially tomatoes and eggplant.

Blood: As blood is the healthiest, most desirable humor, it's good to cultivate it with blood-building foods like spinach, green leafy vegetables, molasses, dark red and blue berries, and various types of meat in moderation. Excessive meat consumption may produce a lot of blood, but it won't be of very high quality, often being too thick, toxic or acidic; blood circulation is also often compromised. Therefore, one shouldn't rely exclusively on meat to build the blood.

Excessive consumption of proteins, rich fatty foods and sweets may lead to Sanguine excesses of the blood, like uremia and gout, diabetes or high cholesterol in those so predisposed. Above all, moderation is needed to avoid the extremes of either overfeeding the body on the one hand or malnourishing it on the other.

Guidelines for Eating

Proper diet involves not just what you eat, but also when, how and how much. The following guidelines should help you establish healthy, sensible eating habits:

1) Never eat when you're tired, angry, upset or worried. Fatigue, negative emotions and stress impair proper digestion.

2) Don't eat unless you're truly hungry. If you're not really hungry, your body isn't really ready to receive the food.

3) Eat your largest meal at midday. When the Sun is at its height, so are our powers of pepsis, or digestion and metabolism.

4) Eat lightly for dinner, at least three hours before retiring. Eating too heavily, too late at night, will leave undigested food to putrefy in the gut and disturb sound sleep, as well as digestion.

5) A little light exercise before meals stimulations the appetite and digestion. It does this by consuming residual humoral superfluities.

6) Drink the most water between meals; sip while you sup. Drinking too much water with meals dilutes the digestive juices, but small amounts will moisten the food and lubricate its passage down the gullet.

7) Don't overeat. Never fill your stomach past three-quarters full. Always leave some space for air, so that your stomach has some working room.

8) Chew your food well before swallowing. Digestion begins in the mouth, by masticating the food and mixing it with saliva.

9) Eat in good company; make meals a happy, joyful occasion. Excessive pensiveness and melancholy ruin digestion.

10) Never eat on the run. Always take the time to digest your food properly. Anxiety and stress interfere with proper digestion.

Moderation in Diet

In dietary matters, Avicenna believed, above all, in moderation and common sense. He believed in avoiding extremes of all kinds. Excess and immoderation in diet are of course harmful, but so is excessive restriction of diet, because the organism bears transgressions of it with more difficulty then a diet that is a little bit more flexible and liberal.

In diet, a distinction must be made between diets that are specifically directed towards some healing goal, versus one's regular diet. Therapeutic or cleansing diets must be more restricted, but excessive restriction is not advisable in one's regular diet.

Exercise and rest

To remain healthy, the organism needs adequate exercise and physical activity to stay in shape. It also needs adequate rest and sleep to allow the regenerative processes time to restore its vital reserves. Optimum health depends on finding the right balance between exercise and rest.

Exercise is a vigorous form of physical activity; however, not all physical activity qualifies as exercise. How do we distinguish between the two?

Exercise is vigorous physical activity, but vigorousness is relative. What may be vigorous activity for some may not be for others.

The criterion for determining what is vigorous activity or exercise for any given individual lies in the respiration. What alters or increases his/her respiratory rate is defined as exercise for that individual; what doesn't, isn't.

Along with the respiratory rate, the pulse rate also increases. The degree of vigor or strenuousness of any exercise workout for a given individual can be measured by how much it raises his/her pulse rate above the normal resting rate.

The Effects and Benefits of Exercise

The physical body and all its constituent parts are kept in shape by regularly performing the functions for which they were designed. In other words: If you don't use it, you lose it.

Persian Medicine recognizes several important effects and benefits of exercise, which are as follows:

By increasing the pulse and respiratory rate, exercise gives a thorough workout to the Vital Faculty, enabling it to become more powerful, energetic and efficient. The increased supply of fresh blood and its life giving pneuma improves the health and functioning of the entire organism.

Exercise tones and conditions the physical body. It enables parts that would otherwise become too soft and flabby, like the muscles, to attain the right tone and firmness, while enabling parts that would otherwise become too stiff and rigid, like the tendons and joints, to maintain the desired suppleness and flexibility.

Exercise dilates and opens the various channels, ducts and vessels of the organism, like the blood vessels and capillaries, and cleanses them of accretions and accumulations of morbid wastes, humors or toxins that may be obstructing them.

Exercise cleanses the organism of superfluous or morbid humors and neutralizes toxins, chiefly by metabolizing and consuming them. In so doing, it awakens the appetite and prepares the organism to receive, digest and metabolize more nourishment.

Exercise lightens the body, aids in weight loss, makes the body nimbler and agile, and improves the reflexes. It also makes the mind more focused and alert.

Exercise, done appropriately and in moderation, will produce all these benefits and more. Excessive or abusive exercise, however, produces exhaustion and fatigue, and is destructive of these ends. A program of physical conditioning should be undertaken gradually, step by step; physical conditioning doesn't happen overnight, and the organism should never be pushed beyond what it is conditioned to handle. Push your body too hard in exercise, and you run the risk of injury.

Varieties and Forms of Exercise

Any vigorous physical activity qualifies as exercise. Heavy physical labor at one's work is also exercise. Or, exercise may be undertaken purely as exercise alone.

There are many forms of exercise, involving a wide variety of movements - slow or swift, gentle or vigorous, continuous or intermittent. Different exercises work different parts or the body, with some focusing on specific parts and others involving more or less the whole body.

Movements may either be active, initiated by the exerciser himself, or passive, arising from without. Sailing and horseback riding are examples of exercises involving a lot of passive movements. Even massage can be seen as a form of passive exercise.

Various exercises can be recommended or prescribed for various conditions, just like any drug or medication.

Exercise and the Four Temperaments

We all need some form of exercise to maintain our health. To ensure that we will continue to exercise on a regular basis, the form of exercise should preferably be one that's appealing to us, and will hold our interest.

Each one of the Four Temperaments has its own particular exercise personality, involving different motivations for exercising, as well as an attraction to different forms of exercise. The astute physician or personal trainer will take these factors of personal temperament into account when designing an exercise program for a patient or client.

The Choleric individual is a natural athlete or sportsman, due to his active, driven, competitive nature. Since he tends to push himself to extremes, he needs to be cautioned not to overdo exercise, particularly when he is out of shape, and run the risk of injury. Choleric are attracted to extreme sports and those involving plenty of thrills and speed. Racing, athletic competitions, and martial arts are also appealing.

The Sanguine individual is an artiste and team player when it comes to exercise. They're not as aggressive or competitive as the Choleric type, and seek out sports involving a lot of grace and finesse. Needing a lot of social interaction, they are natural team players, and excel in team sports. Sanguine undertake exercise in the pursuit of art, beauty and perfection, or to find more joy, happiness and social satisfaction in being active.

The Melancholic individual is drawn to sports of skill, like tennis, or to sports of endurance and efficiency, like long distance running. Sports that get one out in nature help to ground Melancholic and relieve a lot of nervous stress and anxiety. The Melancholic type has certain competitiveness, but it's not as intense or driven as that of the Choleric; rather, it's more of an inner competitiveness that pits self against self to attain new heights of skill, efficiency, performance and endurance.

The Phlegmatic individual is the most passive of all the temperaments, and the least inclined to physical activity. They prefer to exercise the option not to exercise! Still, Phlegmatic can be induced to do the gentler, more appealing forms of exercise if they understand and appreciate the benefits involved. Exercises involving a lot of passive movement, like sailing and horseback riding, are naturals, as are romantic activities. Aquatic sports like swimming diving put Phlegmatic in their element.

The Necessity of Rest

Although most people don't get enough exercise, it is possible to get too much. The signs and symptoms of too much exercise are as follows:

- Fatigue, exhaustion and prostration, especially in the hips and loins.
- Sore, tense or burning muscles; stiff or aching joints
- Frequent or undue sprains, strains or injuries.
- A weak or impaired digestion.
- Inability to relax or unwind; insomnia and loss of sleep.
- Excessive thirst, dehydration
- A dry, withered or emaciated appearance, sunken eyes and temples, hollow cheeks.

Getting adequate rest as well as exercise and physical activity help to keep the two halves of the nervous system - sympathetic and parasympathetic - in balance. It also ensures the thoroughness, vigor and integrity of the digestive and metabolic functions.

Sleep and Wakefulness

Balancing the Daily Cycle

Closely related to the essential factor of Exercise and Rest is that of Sleep and Wakefulness; both help us to maintain a balance in our daily routine and activities.

The Nature of Sleep and Wakefulness

The ancient Iranians were great believers in the restorative power of sleep and rest. Sleep is necessary to allow the anabolic processes the opportunity to restore and regenerate the organism and its vitality.

What sleep does for the body, dreams do for the mind. Dreams enable the mind to regenerate itself and work off all the stresses, problems and tensions of the proceeding day.

When we get sleepy, sweet, Hot, moist Sanguine vapors rise from the heart to the head, and one starts to yawn, sigh and get drowsy. Sleep then starts to overcome us, and the senses start to interiorize; we close our eyes and fall asleep. As the quiescence of sleep deepens, the Sanguine hot starts to cool off, the metabolism slows down, and the circulation interiorizes to hot the body's core. And so, the nature of sleep is cold, wet and Phlegmatic.

Wakefulness has the opposite nature. Its activity is Hot, and in consuming the nutritive and caloric reserves of the organism, wakefulness is Dry. This gives wakefulness a Choleric nature and temperament. Wakefulness is like a flame that consumes the vital nutritive reserves of the organism.

To remain healthy, we need to maintain a balance between Phlegmatic sleep and Choleric wakefulness. Excessive sleep and somnolence makes one too sluggish and phlegmatic. Excessive wakefulness makes us too tense, hyperactive and Choleric. Excessive sleep breeds more Phlegmatic somnolence; excessive wakefulness breeds more Choleric restless activity. And so, a vicious cycle is created.

The nature of sleep is basically the same as that of rest, except that it is deeper and more profound. And the nature of wakefulness is basically the same as that of exercise, except not so vigorous and active.

Sleep is restorative and anabolic. The more healing, growing and regenerative work the organism needs to do, the more sleep it will need. Children and youths, whose bodies are still growing, need more sleep than adults, who have stopped growing, since growth is anabolic.

Constitutional Temperament and Sleep

The more inherent moisture and Radical Moisture you have in your constitutional makeup, the better you will be able to sleep. And so, the wet or moist temperaments - Sanguine and Phlegmatic - are generally the soundest sleepers.

Of all the Four Temperaments, the Phlegmatic temperament - the most passive, and the wettest and most anabolic - is generally the heaviest sleeper. They may even be prone to excessive sleep and somnolence. They also tend to be the heaviest snorers, since the great inherent moisture of their constitutions greatly relaxes the tone of the soft palate, producing excessive snoring.

In the Sanguine temperament, which is moderately moist, and not as wet and anabolic as the Phlegmatic, sleep is sound and balanced, but not excessive. There may be some snoring, but it, too is not excessive.

Insomnia and sleep disorders tend to occur most frequently in the two dry temperaments - Choleric and Melancholic. However, the two differ in their respective patterns of sleep disturbance.

The Choleric pattern is to have no trouble falling asleep, but to then suffer from restless or fitful sleep, tossing and turning all night. Choleric may wake up in the early morning, between 2 and 3 AM, and have a hard time going back to sleep.

The Melancholic pattern is to have a hard time falling asleep, and then not sleep very deeply or soundly even when they do sleep. Melancholic also have a tendency to wake up too early in the morning, thus robbing them of a full night's sleep. Insomnia is most common in Melancholic, who also tends to be the lightest sleepers.

Insomnia and sleep disturbances can also arise from acquired conditions and aggravations of humor and temperament, usually of a Choleric or Melancholic nature. Cholerically, digestive disturbances, generally of a bilious nature, can disturb sleep from eating too heavily for dinner, and too late at night or too soon before retiring. Melancholically, staying up too late at night, or not eating regularly or sensibly for adequate nourishment, can lead to insomnia and sleep disturbances. Excessive anxiety and stress, as well as the abuse of caffeine and other stimulants, can also cause sleep disturbances.

Retention and Evacuation of wastes

It's impossible to live without generating wastes. That's the nature of metabolism, or pepsis, through which the Innate Heat acts on the physical substance of the body and the nutrients it consumes.

The lighter, subtler wastes like exhalation and insensible transpiration are constantly escaping from our bodies, due to the action of the Innate Heat on the substance of the organism. Because these effluents are constantly escaping from the body and depleting its substance, we need to eat and drink to sustain ourselves.

The heavier, denser wastes like urine and feces tend to have the opposite problem: they can get too stuck or congested, and not be eliminated in a prompt, efficient manner. Their undue retention can be just as problematic as their excessive or premature evacuation, if not more so, and can clog the organism and impede its functioning.

And so, the right balance between waste retention and waste evacuation is essential for good hygiene and optimum health. The excessive or premature evacuation of wastes drains the organism of valuable fluids and nutrients that should have been reabsorbed. Excessive waste retention clogs or poisons the organism with toxins in a state called autointoxication.

Both extremes of excessive retention or excessive evacuation of wastes can pose serious threats to life and health. But on the whole, excessive waste retention is much more common and pervasive. Therefore, essential waste management is mainly focused on encouraging the prompt, efficient elimination of wastes on a daily basis, and the therapeutic evacuation of wastes to remedy chronic or excessive retention.

The Four Principle Wastes

There are four principle waste products of the body, each of which corresponds to a different element. The physician, as well as the individual interested in health and longevity must be skilled in the proper management of each.

Exhalation, or the Outbreath - AIR

Exhalation, or the outbreath, is the waste product of the Vital Faculty, the exhaust of cellular metabolism. It's expelled by the lungs, which both inhale fresh air and exhale old, stale air through the process of gas exchange.

For breathing to be healthy, inhalation and exhalation must be balanced. If exhalation exceeds inhalation, there will be gasping, dyspnea and shortness of breath. If inhalation exceeds exhalation, there will be a suffocating, stuffy feeling in the chest and much wheezing, yawning or sighing. Because gas exchange is reciprocal, an excess of either exhalation or inhalation will inhibit the other.

If inhalation is deficient and exhalation excessive, lung and breathing capacity must be increased through gentle aerobic exercise, proper nutrition to build the blood, and herbal tonics for the lungs.

If exhalation is deficient and inhalation excessive, it generally indicates insufficient exercise, which has allowed old, stale air and carbon dioxide to build up in the lungs, and in the blood; exercise more, and stay active. Also, a lot of people are very shallow breathers, and allow a lot of old, stale air to build up in the lungs; to remedy this, do yogic breathing exercises.

The outbreath contains not just old, stale air, but also residual or superfluous moisture, as well as the gaseous vapors of other humors. If these get offensive, a condition known as halitosis, or bad breath, develops. Most often, bad breath results from excessive putrid, acrid or sour humors in the stomach.

Sweat

Sweat is the next subtlest of the four principle wastes. It belongs to the Fire element, and is the body's main way of cooling itself and releasing excessive heat.

Sweat is both the gross, visible perspiration that usually happens only in hot weather, or with vigorous exercise and activity; and the subtle insensible transpiration that's always being released by the skin due to the action of the Innate Heat. Because we're always sweating, in one form or another, we must drink fluids to replenish this loss.

The sweat, especially insensible transpiration, has a close relationship with the exhalation; both eliminate excess moisture and subtle vaporous humors from the body. Together, the lungs and skin form the surface complex, which is the body's first line of defense against colds, flu and exogenous or environmental pathogenic factors.

When the skin is attacked by a chilly draft, the pores close up to protect against the invasion, and all sweating, both sensible and insensible, stops. The fluids that would have been sweated out through the skin back up into the lungs, producing congestion and coughing.

Sweat also has a close relationship with urine, the body's other form of liquid waste; in its chemical composition, and sweat resembles a very dilute form of urine. Those with weak, hypofunctioning kidneys will often sweat easily or excessively; the organism is trying to release the wastes it would have eliminated in the urine via the sweat.

If the Vital Force and Thymus are deficient, there will often be a light, furtive sweat that's always present, even without hot weather or vigorous exercise. The body's immune shield isn't vigorous enough to prevent the sweat from escaping. Other deficiency types of sweating are caused by nervous exhaustion, or neurasthenia; prostration, or marasmus; and various consumptive conditions. Excessive sweating can be stopped with anhydrotics.

The health conscious individual is always mindful of the condition of the skin and its pores. If the pores have been unduly opened by a hot bath, vigorous exercise, and the like, he/she guards against chills.

Diaphoresis, or sweating, is one of the Six Essential Purification Methods of Persian Medicine. It cleanses the blood by releasing toxins via the sweat. Sweating can be enhanced or provoked to treat various conditions, like colds and flu or skin conditions, by drinking hot diaphoretic herb teas like Peppermint or Elder flower, or by massaging the body with medicated oils and sweating in a sauna. Sweating is a good preparatory therapy for deeper forms of cleansing.

When there's an excess of morbid humors and toxins, body odor can become overpowering or offensive. Toxic sweat can also burn and sting. Persian Medicine recommends the use of various natural essences and aromatics to impart a pleasant odor to the body, but disapproves of deodorants which inhibit perspiration, which is a natural, cleansing bodily function.

Urine

Urine is the body's main liquid waste. Water soluble wastes and superfluities in the blood plasma are eliminated from the body via the urine. Urine production involves not just the Water element, but also the Fire element as the Metabolic Heat working through the kidneys to ripen and eliminate wastes via the urine.

The main waste product in the urine is urea, a protein byproduct that colors the urine yellow. The urine also eliminates excesses or superfluities of fluids and electrolytes. Through selective elimination and reabsorption via metabolism and filtration, the kidneys balance and purify the fluids in the bloodstream.

The kidneys, being a metabolic organ of the Natural Faculty, are greatly impacted by what we eat and drink. For optimum urinary function and health, the diet must be watched closely in the following areas:

Water and Fluids: Water and fluid consumption should be ample but not excessive, and adjusted according to endogenous constitutional factors as well as exogenous factors of weather, climate and activity level. 1500 +_500 cc per day is the standard, with cold weather or climate, a moist constitution and sedentariness decreasing the need, and a hot weather or climate, a dry constitution and vigorous activity increasing it.

The water drunk should also be pure. It should not be ice cold, since ice cold drinks injure the kidneys, depleting them of the Metabolic Heat they need to properly process and ripen the urine. Drinking ice cold drinks can also aggravate cramps and spasms, as well as urinary imbalances of either excessive or deficient urination.

The excessive consumption of fruit juices, as well as coffee and caffeinated tea, over stimulations the kidneys and is excessively diuretic. Certain herb teas can be drunk liberally throughout the day like water, to heal and balance the urinary tract.

Sugar and Salt: Excessive salt consumption weakens the kidneys, favors edema and water retention, and the retention of wastes that can aggravate uremia, gout, hypertension, and arthritic conditions. Excessive consumption of sugar and sweets also weakens the kidneys, especially in those with diabetic tendencies.

Fruit and Vegetables: Eating plenty of fresh fruits and vegetables is necessary to cleanse and alkalinize the blood, which aids kidney function. Excessive fruit consumption, especially to the detriment of vegetables, has an overly diuretic effect that weakens the kidneys. Certain fruits, like watermelons, are very diuretic.

Meat and Protein: Excessive meat consumption overburdens the liver and kidneys with too much uric acid, and can aggravate conditions like uremia and gout. Other types of protein, if consumed in great excess, can also injure the kidneys and urinary tract function.

Fat: Excessive fat consumption is bad for the circulatory system, as we all know. Since the circulatory system and Vital Faculty are closely connected with the kidneys and urinary function, what injures the former will also injure the latter.

Exercise, activity and lifestyle factors are also important in maintaining urinary health. Basically, whatever causes undue fatigue, stress or prostration is bad, since the kidneys and urinary tract are energetically linked to the Vital Faculty through the adrenal glands, which sit on top of them. Excessive sexual activity can also drain the kidneys and urinary tract, especially in men.

Diuresis, which is Stimulating or provoking urination, is one of the Six Essential Purification Methods of Persian Medicine.

Since uric acid is yellow, hot and caustic, Persian Medicine considers it to be Choleric in nature. And so, diuresis is the main hygienic therapy for removing toxins from the blood, especially hot, caustic Choleric toxins that irritate and inflame.

Diuretics are herbs or medicines that stimulation or provoke urination. They are indicated in all conditions involving deficient or defective urinary function, which include urinary tract infections, edema and water retention, arthritis and rheumatism, uremia and gout, diabetes and metabolic disorders, and certain rashes and skin conditions. Many herbs and medicines have either stronger or weaker diuretic actions, each with its own particular nature and indications in treating the above conditions.

The whole secret to urinary health lies in keeping a balance: between retention and elimination, between inherent functional vitality of the kidneys versus exogenous purification and Stimulation.

The Stool

The stool or feces, also called the Alvine Discharge, being the body's main solid waste, is also the one most prone to stagnation and excessive retention. Although excessive or premature evacuation of the stool can be dangerous, even life-threatening, excessive retention is much more common.

Excessive or premature evacuation of the stool is called diarrhea, and can have many causes. Acute diarrhea is usually caused by infection or inflammation, and can be seen as the protective response of the organism to get rid of noxious, irritating or offensive matter. If acute diarrhea is excessive or severe, the greatest threat to life and health is from dehydration, or the loss of valuable fluids and electrolytes. Most chronic forms of diarrhea are due to digestive atony and a deficient Metabolic Heat of digestion that fails to reabsorb sufficient fluids and electrolytes, making the stool loose and watery.

Constipation is the root cause of more chronic and degenerative conditions than just about any other hygienic problem. These conditions include: arthritis, rheumatism, acid reflux, intestinal obstruction, insomnia, bad breath, headaches, dizziness, sore throat, sciatica, lumbago and hemorrhoids, to mention only a few.

The colon can be compared to the roots of a large tree. Old retained wastes and fecal matter putrefy in the colon, which then reabsorbs these toxins back into the organism, causing a condition known as autointoxication or alimentary toxemia.

Those warning of the dangers of constipation and its involvement in chronic disease say, "Death begins in the colon." Those preferring to focus on the positive say, "Life begins with a clean colon."

The first line of treatment for constipation is dietary. Unless the right dietary changes are made, relief of constipation will only be partial, temporary and unsatisfactory.

If none of these other laxatives work, the last resort is to use Persian Medicine plant laxatives, which are also called purgatives. But their action is very harsh, and the risk of abuse and dependency is high.

Excessive or repeated strong, harsh Stimulation of the bowels can drain their inherent vitality and function. This can create a dependency on harsh stimulant laxatives.

Besides laxatives and purgatives, Persian Medicine also uses other therapies to cleanse the colon, where appropriate and indicated. These chiefly consist of various types of enemas; colonic irrigation could also be included as its modern version. Laxatives and purgatives as well as enemas and colonics are all included under Purgation therapy as one of the Six Essential Purification Methods of Persian Medicine. Enemas and colonics are called procured evacuations, because a physician or therapist usually performs them.

Toxins tend to build up more quickly in the organism, and bowel function tends to become more sluggish as we age. And so, it's a good idea to undertake a cleansing regime with enemas and colonics about once or twice a year, especially in middle age and beyond.

The Minor Wastes

The organism eliminates other wastes besides the four principle ones. These include smegma, ear wax, tooth tartar, tongue coatings, sebaceous secretions, pus, and vaginal secretions. These are studied carefully by the Iranian Physician, because they yield valuable clues as to what's going on in the body. Basically, the organism will try to eliminate accumulations of toxins and morbid, superfluous humors, wherever they may be, through the most convenient route, or orifice available to it. What the organism is eliminating spontaneously through these exudations and secretions will tell the physician a lot about which toxins and morbid humors need to be reduced, cleansed, or brought back into balance.

Mental Hygiene

The ancient Iranians considered the health of the mind to be just as important as the health of the body. Their ideal of health was expressed in the maxim, "A sound mind in a healthy body." Persian Medicine is holistic in that it views the mind and body as being interconnected, and essentially one.

This last of the Six Essential Principles can be seen as the psychological counterpart of Exercise and Rest; it's Somtimes called Psychic Activity and Rest. Although it's subtle and invisible, the activity or life of the mind and Psychic Faculty is just as important to our health and vitality as our physical activities and lifestyle.

The ancient Iranians saw the life of the mind and psyche in terms of the Four Elements and their associated temperaments. For mental and emotional health, moderation and balance, or a good mixture of all the temperaments and their associated emotions was essential. No emotion is inherently good or evil, but it can become negative and destructive if overly indulged in. Each person, according to his/her constitutional nature and temperament, is predisposed to emotional excesses of his/her dominant temperament.

Proper management of the mind and emotions comes from self-knowledge and from understanding the underlying psychological dynamics of one's prevailing nature. Each of the Four Temperaments has its own inherent strengths, as well as its own weaknesses, or shadow side.

Managing the Choleric Emotions

The negative Choleric emotions are anger, rage, impatience, irritability, frustration, jealousy, criticalness, contentiousness and treachery. Fire can be very destructive, as can be these negative Choleric emotions; either they explode, causing sudden chaos and violent destruction, or they slowly eat away at one's guts, like a festering tumor or ulcer.

Properly channeled and directed, Fire can be very powerful, dynamic and transformative. The positive Choleric emotions are those that motivate and inspire us to take action, fight the good fight, and achieve great things: courage, boldness, fearlessness, valor and ambition. Yet even these need to be tempered by reason and reflection, otherwise they can become too reckless and impulsive: discretion is the better part of valor.

When positive, constructive outlets for Fire's energy and dynamism are blocked or obstructed, we run into the negative Choleric emotions. If the obstruction is acute, we get explosions of anger and rage. These paroxysms of excess gall and biliousness explode from the liver into the head, causing headaches, migraines, apoplexy and sore, bloodshot eyes. The more chronic negative Choleric emotions like jealousy are held in the epigastrium, and slowly eat away at our guts and vitals.

The positive Choleric emotions like courage and fearlessness are held in the heart, and serve to strengthen and expand the Vital Spirits. They spur us on to victory, and strengthen our energy, determination and resolve.

In between the resignation of defeat and the exaltation of victory lies the anger band, a critical zone that can go either way, depending on how we handle it. Being able to successfully rechanneled one's anger and aggression into victory requires considerable detachment, mental clarity and resourcefulness, but it can be done.

Often, anger can be a violent reaction against something that subliminally frightens or terrifies us, or paralyzes us with fear, hopelessness and resignation. We must put our finger on these hidden fears before we can take steps to resolve them positively.

Whether positive or negative, powerful Choleric emotions involve great stress and struggle, and can be quite draining energetically. We need to find ways of chilling out, disengaging from it all, and recharging our energies. The negative Choleric emotions, whether acute or chronic, can be very disturbing and destructive of inner peace and tranquility.

Perhaps the most pernicious threat of the negative Choleric emotions is that, if denied an outlet, they will turn inwards to "implode", or destroy the individual himself. Choleric tend to be contentious, critical and often unforgiving; they must learn how to be more tolerant and accepting, and to forgive themselves, as well as others.

Managing the Sanguine Emotions

The Sanguine temperament is the most desirable of them all. Similarly, the Sanguine emotions like joy, euphoria, expansiveness, exaltation and all forms of pleasure are what we all live for. Many of us can't get enough of these emotions, and may even feel shortchanged in their fulfillment.

But even these most desirable Sanguine emotions have their shadow side, which results from their excess, perversion, or abuse. These include lust, gluttony, indulgence, debauchery and jaded appetites. One can even lose oneself in too much joy.

The desirable Sanguine emotions are all exhilarating and expansive, but overexpansion can dissipate and weaken the character. We all know of the spoiled brat who has never had to endure any deprivation, discipline or hardship.

How do we maintain a sense of self, character and integrity, and not lose ourselves when great joys or pleasures come our way? This is precisely why Persian Medicine considers moderation and the Golden Mean to be so important. So enjoy pleasures responsibly, and always with a sense of equanimity and self-respect.

To keep the Sanguine joys and indulgences within their proper bounds, Persian Medicine advocates temperance. Temperance means tempering or balancing something with its complementary opposite - in this case, a pragmatic, prudent sense of duty, responsibility and the necessities of life. These limitations and restrictions must be voluntary and self-imposed.

With the ancient Iranians, temperance was motivated by more pragmatic concerns for the greater dignity, integrity, self-control and happiness of the individual over the long term.

Managing the Melancholic Emotions

Because the Melancholic temperament is the least desirable in terms of health, it follows that the Melancholic emotions are also the least desirable. The word melancholy has become synonymous with depression and the blues.

In general, Melancholic emotions have a consolidating, constricting effect that favors sobriety, reflection and withdrawal. They also tend to be heavy, somber and grave.

Some Melancholic emotions, like caution, prudence and realism, in the proper mean and measure, can have constructive applications, and keep the Sanguine joys and indulgences within the proper bounds. Equanimity is maintained by never forgetting sorrow, even in the midst of great joy, and never forgetting hardship and deprivation, even in the midst of success and plenty.

Other Melancholic emotions, like loneliness, depression and grief, can have much more negative consequences, especially if prolonged or excessive. There are no bad emotions, and all of us have to experience these sometime in our lives, but problems arise when we can't process them properly, and get chronically stuck in them.

Some of the most pernicious Melancholic emotions are perversions or aggravations of more positive ones, which can have a constructive purpose. Pragmatism and realism can degenerate into caution and prudence can degenerate into misanthropy.

Melancholic emotions like pensiveness, moodiness and worry will ruin proper digestion, and lead to the nervous, colicky digestive complaints that Melancholic are famous for.

There are certain dangers or negative side effects that those who overindulge in Melancholic emotions are prone to:

First of all, they make the individual too withdrawn, isolating him/her from healthy communication and social contact with others. The person retreats into their own little world of worries and anxieties. Secondly, they can make many people too rigid or dogmatic in their thinking. The spontaneity needed to enjoy life and take it as it comes is also often ruined. Melancholic types can also get too analytical, and rationalize away their emotions.

Managing the Phlegmatic Emotions

The greatest things about the Phlegmatic mentality and outlook on life, from which arise the Phlegmatic emotions, are a patient, devotional nature; a deep, abiding faith; and a remarkable good-naturedness. Phlegmatic are slow to anger and quick to forgive, as water dissolves all hardness and smooth away all rough edges.

But since Water is also the most passive element and the greatest absorber of energy, the greatest weakness of the Phlegmatic emotional nature is its tendency towards passivity, which can plunge into a deep torpor of sluggishness and indifference. Phlegmatic need to learn how to rise up, take charge, and make the quantum leap from thought to action.

Emotional subjectivity and receptivity is also a great weak point. Excessive subjectivity makes it hard to make objective, rational decisions, as Phlegmatic find it hard to get the necessary detachment and perspective. Excessive receptivity makes one hypersensitive, overwhelmed, and emotionally shell-shocked, and unable to respond effectively to life. Raising your level of awareness is always a good thing, but increasing your sensitivity is not always good.

Heightened subjectivity and sensitivity, plus a heightened suggestibility and receptivity to subconscious influences, tend to weaken the power of the will in Phlegmatic types. This also heightens passivity and an inability to take effective, decisive action. Phlegmatic also tend to be creatures of habit.

The Phlegmatic emotional mindset is the perfect complement and antidote to the Choleric. Phlegmatic passivity tames the wild recklessness and impulsiveness of the Choleric nature, and Phlegmatic receptivity and subjectivity soften and restrain the excessive willfulness that Choleric are prone to. Above all, Choleric need to learn patience, tolerance, faith, forgiveness and compassion, which the Phlegmatic nature has in abundance.

Perhaps the most healing and transformative Phlegmatic emotions are empathy and compassion. Compassion means, "suffering with" - the ability to put yourself in another person's shoes, to identify with and feel their pain and suffering. This leads to a great emotional catharsis and cleansing, and a profound transformation as we realize universal solidarity with the human condition. This emotional cleansing or catharsis is a manifestation of the Expulsive Virtue of the Water element. Compassion is also the basis for many of the world's great religions.

Closely related to compassion are the Phlegmatic emotions of love and devotion; their aim is to soften a hardened heart, to make it more receptive to inspiration and healing. Love takes no offense, accepts and endures all things, is slow to anger, and eventually conquers all. Devotional paths to God are based on a personal love for and relationship with, a personification of divinity. They are favored by those of a sentimental nature and Phlegmatic temperament, and are the perfect antidote for those who feel overwhelmed by a sense of harsh impersonality and indifference in the universe. Religious devotion is indeed an eternal spring of living waters that can sate the spiritual thirst of man.

Balancing the Emotions

It should be clear by now that the best way to manage or remedy the negative emotions of one temperament is to counterbalance or temper them with the positive emotions of its opposite yet complementary temperament, backed up by that contrary temperament's philosophical mindset. And so:

Choleric anger, frustration, irritability, impatience and intolerance must be remedied by Phlegmatic peace and tranquility, faith and tolerance, and devotional surrender to a Higher Power.

Sanguine sensuality, indulgence, euphoria and immoderation must be remedied with Melancholic realism, prudence and temperance.

Melancholic austerity, wearisomeness, guilt, depression, rigidity and withdrawal must be remedied with a Sanguine appreciation of the joys and pleasures of life advocated by the Epicurean philosophy.

Phlegmatic passivity, lethargy and resignation must be remedied with Choleric action, ambition and drive, and the philosophy of rugged individualism that underlies it.

The proper balance and regulation of our emotional life is an important part of our daily hygiene. It's important not only to the health of the mind, but, as we have just seen, to the health of the body, and all its internal organs.

Cleanliness is Health

The ancient Iranians had the wisdom and insight to know that bodily cleanliness was an essential component of good hygiene and good health.

Bathing is a way of caring for and loving the body by taking good care of it. This ran counter to the Church's prevailing attitude of ascetic denial and despising of the body and its needs.

Steam Baths or Hammams

In these baths, first, you are given a towel, some soap, a key, and a cloth skirt, or wrap. You enter a private cubicle and undress, wrapping yourself in the wrap.

Then, you enter the main room of the bath. You are doused with water, and then rubbed with mitts of coarse muslin cloth to rub off the residual dead skin.

Next follows a thorough sudsing and rubdown with soap, worked into a profuse lather. Then, you are dowsed again and rinsed of the suds. A second sudsing and lathering follows, followed by a second rinse.

Then, you soak in a hot tub, or lie on a hot marble slab to relax and chill out. If you wish, you may receive a massage with fragrant, scented medicinal oils.

When you come out, you feel thoroughly refreshed, revitalized and thoroughly clean.

Fasting and purification (The Physician Within)

"Everyone has a physician inside him or her; we just have to help it in its work. The natural healing force within each one of us is the greatest force in getting well. Our food should be our medicine. Our medicine should be our food. But to eat when you are sick is to feed your sickness." *Avicenna*

When an animal is sick, its natural instinct is to refuse food. When the crisis is over, and the internal healing work has been accomplished, the appetite will return naturally, of its own accord.

The human organism also has a fasting instinct, just like that of other animals. Evolutionary adaptation has made our bodies very efficient at storing energy reserves, and drawing upon them when food supplies are scarce.

Fasting is as old as mankind, perhaps even older. As far back as historians can see, men have been fasting for one reason or another. It seems to be a universal practice.

The ancient Iranians were great believers in fasting. Avicenna advocated it, as is shown in the above quotation.

Purposes and Benefits of Fasting

Basically, there are two kinds of purposes or objectives for fasting. Men fast for either spiritual or physical reasons or both are equally valid.

Spiritually, fasting helps us transcend our addiction and attachment to food, and to realize that man doesn't live by bread alone. The mind gets clearer, and spiritual awareness deepens. Freed from having to satisfy physical hunger, one can then turn one's attention to feeding the mind and spirit. Spiritual masters wouldn't admit any disciple into their higher teachings unless they had first purified themselves through fasting.

Physically, fasting enables the organism to detoxify and clean house. Because the vast majority of diseases are caused by autointoxication, fasting has wide-ranging therapeutic benefits. It also gives the digestive organs a much needed rest.

For all fevers and diseases in the acute crisis stage, Avicenna prescribed either a strict fast with nothing but water or medicinal teas, or a very slender liquid diet. Fasting is also recommended for colds and flu, arthritis and rheumatism, digestive complaints, and all humoral and metabolic disorders.

Scientific experiments conducted on laboratory mice have shown that severe restriction of caloric intake greatly extends their lifespan. Since this is basically what fasting is, fasting holds great promise for life extension.

The Physiology of Fasting

As long as we're alive, the Innate Heat, or metabolic fire, is always active. And as long as this metabolic fire is burning, it must consume something for fuel.

Normally, this Innate Heat or metabolic fire is fed by nutrients from the food we eat. But when we fast, we cut off this outer supply of fuel, and the metabolic fire begins to feed on the body's own inner reserves. The body's own Inner Physician is awakened, and the human organism, in its infinite healing wisdom, starts to clean house and burn off the dross.

What is least essential to the life and health of the organism is consumed first, such as toxins, wastes, and superfluous morbid humors. The Inner Physician knows precisely where to go, what to metabolize and eliminate, and how to eliminate it. This is the process of autolysis. In this sense, fasting has been described as an operation without surgery.

Fasting gives your digestive organs a much needed rest. Instead of digesting food, their digestive secretions and enzymes can serve to digest, neutralize and eliminate toxic wastes from the body via the GI tract. Chief among these secretions is bile, which is secreted by the liver and gall bladder.

Depending on where the toxins and morbid humors have been held in the body, they will start to produce various signs and symptoms as this waste is eliminated and passed off:

Head / Brain: headaches, dizziness, vertigo, wooziness, lightheadedness.

Nose, Sinuses: sneezing, runny nose, itching, stinging, post nasal drip.

Throat: soreness or constriction, hoarseness, scratchiness

Lungs: chest congestion, wheezing, phlegm discharges, foul breath odors

Skin: rashes, acne, pustules; excessive or abnormal sweating; strange body odors

Stomach: sour or nervous stomach, stomach cramping, belching, bad breath

Liver: sore eyes, bitter taste in mouth, sallow complexion, pain or distension under the ribs on the right side.

Gall Bladder: colic, spasm, tenderness or pain underneath the liver area.

Intestines: foul smelling gas, cramping, diarrhea, spastic colon or irritable bowel.

Kidneys: low back pain and weakness, fatigue; frequent urination, often urgent; strongly colored or smelling urine.

Generally, the more recently acquired toxins and accumulations of morbid matter will be the first to be passed off, followed by older and more long-standing ones, backtracking in reverse order of acquisition. Also, the day's detoxification tends to start in the morning with head symptoms, and generally works its way down the body.

The cleansing and detoxification symptoms, and the loss of weight and muscle mass, are the most severe and intense for the first three days. Within these first three days, energy levels also tend to be lowest and most problematic. After this initial three-day period, a change happens in the body's internal energy economy, called ketosis, in which the organism switches over to the more efficient burning of its fat reserves to satisfy its basic energy needs. Then, the energy levels get a lot better.

During a fast, the organism detoxifies itself during the night, leaving a thick, foul, bitter tasting residue on the tongue in the morning. Upon arising, it's good to go to the bathroom with a spoon or tongue scraper and scrape this residue off.

Precautions for Fasting

Before fasting, it's good to talk it over with someone who's fasted before, hearing their story, so you have a better idea of what to expect. A short fast of three days or less is a fairly simple affair, and can be undertaken without too much care or concern.

But long fasts, for over three days, are a different matter. For these, it's a good idea to check with your physician to assess whether or not you're able to go through with it physically, especially if you have health conditions like asthma or type 2 diabetes that have compromised your basic health or metabolism. It's also a good idea to have your fasting program designed and monitored by a holistic healthcare professional. One thing that's imperative while fasting is to drink plenty of fluids. These include water, herbal teas and, in the case of juice fasting, fruit and/or vegetable juices. And so, the Expulsive Virtue of the Water element is used to aid the cleansing and detoxification process.

Most of the fasting that was done was water fasting, in which nothing but water was consumed. This is not only the simplest form of fasting, but also the most severe, because it makes stringent demands on the organism to digest and metabolize superfluities and draw on its own internal energy reserves.

Nowadays, water fasting may be alright for short fasts of three days or less, but it's generally not advised for fasts of longer duration. Various abuses prevalent in the modern world, such as environmental pollution; refined, devitalized, nutrient-depleted foods; junk foods and binge eating; and drug and substance abuse have made modern man constitutionally weaker and less resistant to the rigors of intense detoxification.

Before deciding to undertake a long fast, one should get a clean bill of basic health from a physician or holistic healthcare professional. The question is: After prolonged fasting has removed all that is toxic, morbid and superfluous, will you still have the basic constitutional strength and resistance left to sustain yourself through the recuperation and recovery process? Many whose general health condition is too delicate or rundown would be better able to handle an extended fast if they first went on a program of notification and constitutional improvement beforehand.

Types of Fasts and Cleansing Diets

Fasts and cleansing diets are of many different types. They are undertaken for many different purposes and objectives.

A simple fast doesn't exceed more than a day or two in length, and is undertaken when one feels indigestion, lack of appetite, being under the weather, or out of sorts. In its simplest form, it consists merely of skipping a meal, usually dinner. In addition to water, herb teas may be drunk that are specific to the condition you're trying to overcome; with digestion of food no longer necessary, the organism is free to catch up on back healing work. Avicenna prescribed simple fasts in all fevers and acute diseases in the crisis stage.

Juice fasting is the usual modern method for handling fasts of longer duration, where a deeper and more thorough cleansing and detoxification is desired. Fruit and vegetable juices, often diluted 50/50 with pure water, alkalinize the system and speed up detoxification while providing a base level of calories and nutrients to sustain energy; on the other hand, ketosis, or the body's digging into its own fat and energy reserves, isn't as intense. In addition, fruit and vegetable juices, properly chosen, can be therapeutic in many chronic and degenerative conditions, and aid the healing process. In the first two or three days of a juice fast, the bowels are cleansed with enemas or colonics; this greatly decreases the toxic load on the body, and keeps toxins from old fecal wastes retained in the colon from being reabsorbed into the body and the bloodstream.

Cleansing diets involve eating very lightly of food that is very pure, simple, balanced and easy to digest. This provides for the body's basic energy and nutritional needs while allowing cleansing and detoxification to occur. Cleansing diets are very useful for those whose constitutions are too delicate or run down to withstand the quicker, more radical detoxification of a water or juice fast.

By adjusting the ratio of barley to water, or by either straining the barley water or leaving the barley grains in the ptisan, it can be adjusted to virtually any desired consistency. The great value of barley is that it's nourishing, easy to digest, and soothing and emollient to the GI tract, with no residual astringency that might aggravate colic or bloating.

In acute crises and fevers, only the liquid, strained ptisan is used. For ordinary detoxification purposes, a soupy gruel is used. If a broader nutritional base is desired, root or leafy vegetables, sea vegetables, herbs, or beans and pulses can also be cooked in to the ptisan; this also makes for a good transition back to an ordinary diet.

Breaking a Fast

The most critically important part of a fast is how you end it, or break it. Any fool can fast, but breaking it properly is an art, and not so easy. The body must make a gradual, step-by-step transition back to a normal diet. If a prolonged fast isn't broken properly, toxins and fecal matter can recongest the gut, and the bloodstream, and all the benefits of the fast are nullified.

For breaking a fast, ptisan is very useful. On the first day after a prolonged juice fast, drink only the strained barley water. On the second day, a thin, soupy gruel is best, and on the third day, a thicker gruel can be had. On the fourth day, you can cook in lentils and vegetables as well, and on the fifth day, you can go back to your normal diet.

If you can spare the time to do so, spend as much time transitioning back to your normal diet as you did fasting. Remember: The wheels of Nature grind slowly, but very well. If your bowel movements don't return right away, just wait a few days; it takes time for them to be reestablished. Choleric may have to temper their impatience when it comes to breaking a fast if they're not going to nullify all the benefits gained.

The Optimum timing of Fasting

The first rule in timing a fast is that of necessity, and of listening to your body. A fast is indicated whenever toxicity in the body is heading towards a crisis. If symptoms like a cold, poor appetite or indigestion appear, a short, remedial fast is indicated.

When planning a more extensive or prolonged fast, one should pay heed to the season of the year and the phase of the Moon. A prolonged fast should be undertaken in a season in which the weather is neither too hot nor too cold: in the spring, after the last cold snaps of winter have ended; or in the early fall, before the first cold snaps of approaching winter.

Regarding the lunar phases, the waning hemicycle of the Moon favors cleansing and purification, whereas the waxing hemicycle favors recovery and rebuilding after the fast. If you can break the fast around the time of the New Moon, you can utilize the waxing Moon's energy to rebuild.

Fasting and Life Stage

Although a simple remedial fast of skipping a meal or two until your appetite returns is advisable at any age or life stage, the different stages of life differ significantly in their ability to tolerate or handle longer fasts. Children and youths handle fasting the most poorly, because their growing bodies require a richer supply of nutrients. Children and infants tolerate fasting the least, because their bodies are growing the most rapidly.

Pregnant mothers should not fast, because they must eat not just for themselves, but also for the embryo/fetus, which grows the fastest of all.

Young adults may safely undertake short fasts of up to three days, but not much more, unless indicated. That's because their energy and nutritional needs are still considerable.

Those in old age can safely undertake short fasts of up to three days. That's because their constitutions are more delicate, and unable to withstand the rigors of extended fasting.

Those in maturity or middle age are generally the best suited for extended fasting, and are also those who can derive the most benefit from it. After age 40, the metabolism tends to slow down, and doesn't demand or consume as much energy as before. Because the metabolism is slower, toxic residues and morbid humors build up in the system much more quickly, and can be much more problematic. Periodic, judicious fasting during maturity can burn off these toxic residues and morbid humors, thus preventing many degenerative diseases of old age.

Etiology in Persian Medicine

This section on the Etiology in Persian Medicine, the principle of 'cause and effect' is discussed in relation to health maintenance and the cause of disease. The philosophical basis of Persian Medicine provides a strong foundation for both a comprehensive understanding of the different causes of illnesses, and the active maintenance of health. This section looks at causes from different perspectives and direct to the primary causes of all illnesses.

Overview on the Etiology of health and disease

This section discusses Etiology, the study or science of the causes of illnesses.

In Persian Medicine, however the causes of illnesses are also responsible, directly or indirectly for the maintenance of health. It is relatively easy to define illness in terms of tissue or organ malfunction, but defining health is a rather more difficult challenge. Health is a positive, definite concept, not simply the absence of illness.

The practice of Persian Medicine is as relevant to people who are healthy as it is to patients who are ill. The appetite for health is more than simply avoiding illness; it is the desire to pursue a lifestyle which allows the person to function at the optimum, ideal level, and to maintain the physical, mental and spiritual activities which are necessary to get the most out of life. An already healthy person can actively improve his or her physical and mental health.

This section will discuss causes on the assumption that a person is born normal, and without any significant physical or mental abnormality. Persian Medicine strongly believes that everyone has a natural tendency towards health, and that this is the normal condition. The Persian Medicine principle of 'cause and effect' provides insights for both health maintenance and the onset of disease.

Principles of cause and effect

Background

Medical science deals with the human body in both health and disease. It is committed to the identification, isolation and possible elimination of the cause(s) of the illness.

We arrive at a greater understanding of a particular disease if we find out what causes it. This is the science of Etiology. Although the cause may be evident in many diseases, there may be other conditions which may have more obscure causes.

Different circumstances result in a cause being labelled differently. For example, Somtimes one disease causes another disease (as colic can cause convulsions or epilepsy) and Somtimes a symptom becomes the cause for a disease (an acute pain in colic becomes the cause for the occurrence of syncope, or fainting). Similarly, acute pain causes swelling (from the accumulation of matter in response to the area of the pain). Somtimes a condition can be indicative of a cause, a symptom and a disease. For example, a headache caused by a prolonged fever, can leads to meningitis.

Mean of "cause"

In Persian Medicine, cause in the context of medicine is that event, behaviour, or change in the microcosm or macrocosm from which originates the outcome of a certain state of the human body, be it a state of health or disease.

In medical terms, the cause of a disease is a factor associated with the definitive onset of the disease. It can also apply to an injury, or accident. It is different to a risk or pre-disposing factor, which is an attribute of behaviour or habit which makes a person more likely, or probable, to develop a particular illness. Persian

Medicine's understanding of the cause of the disease includes what are generally known as risk factors.

Causes need to fulfil three conditions in order to produce an effect

(a) Sufficient active power

This means that the cause must be able to produce an effect. We don't expect a slight knock to produce a huge bruise

(b) Sufficient receptive power

This means that the body must be able to respond to the cause by reacting appropriately. The biochemical mechanisms responsible for developing an infection, for instance, should be functioning before the infection occurs.

(c) Prolonged contact between the two.

This means that the cause must have time to exert its action. A brief rise in blood pressure, for example, should not cause kidney failure.

Mean of "effect"

An effect is the result of a course of treatment or medical intervention. However, it does not always follow that a course of treatment with a drug, for example, results in an effect which is only due to the drug. There could be a clinical improvement which is due to:

(a) Spontaneous healing or remission.

Spontaneous healing, or remission, is the often sudden but inexplicable recovery from clinical disorders without any real medical intervention. The recovery from the disorder may not be due to the drug or other treatment, but in spite of it. The person's physis is able to restore the internal harmony which is the underlying problem. In fact, more than 80% of clinical disorders improve or completely heal on their own, without any outside intervention.

(b) The placebo response.

A placebo is a therapeutically worthless, inactive, neutral substance made to physically resemble the active drug. A placebo effect is an unanticipated mind-produced response to a placebo. The placebo response would appear to be close or even identical to the physis response. However, as physis transcends the physical, emotional and spiritual dimensions of the person, although it can manifest in one form or another.

Cause and disease

The humoral theory of disease is undoubtedly the most prevalent explanation of disease world-wide. This asserts that an imbalance in a person's humors – hot or cold, moist or dry – is responsible for disease.

Persian Medicine recognises that changes in a person's humoral balance are the underlying cause of specific diseases, and that this is brought about by non-adherence of the lifestyle factors.

Let us discuss the concept of cause resulting in a state of disease, by considering the following case history:

Mr X., aged 60, somewhat overweight, smokes 30 cigarettes a day, drinks quite heavily, exercises very occasionally, and is a mild type 2 diabetic. One day, after a difficult time in the office, and when having an argument with his daughter in the evening, he suffers a non-fatal heart attack.

The question is: What caused X's myocardial infarction?

- Was it one of the several risk factors (smoking, overweight, binge drinking, and glucose intolerance) for atherosclerosis he possesses?

▪ Was it the emotional stress brought about by his confrontation with his daughter?

▪ Was it the atherosclerotic plaque in his coronary artery, preventing adequate blood flow to the heart muscle?

▪ Was it a blood clot, formed in the leg, but carried to the heart by the bloodstream, where it became stuck in an artery?

▪ Was it his sedentary lifestyle?

▪ Was it his genetic makeup?

There is, in this case, a series of possible causes, any one of which could be responsible for his heart attack.

Types of causes

According to Ibn Sina, there are four different kinds of causes:

• **Material causes** – substances (structures) upon which health and disease depend.

In this case, this would include disharmony in circulating lipids and glucose that existed in X, ulimately as a result of a poor diet. The term material cause would invariably refer to foods and derivatives – that is, associated with the humors or body fluids.

• **Formal causes** – those which maintain or alter the body.

With X, this would be his constitution or genetic make-up, or temperament, and its failure to prevent the build-up of atherosclerotic plaques in his coronary arteries (inherited) associated with the temperament of the person.

• **Efficient causes** – the effect on temperament from the environment or lifestyle factors.

For X, this would mean his sedentary lifestyle, which causes an imbalance in humors, which leads to structural changes in the heart's arteries. The heart attack would be triggered by the emotional stress of the argument with his daughter this is the interaction between man and the environment associated with the lifestyle factors.

• **Final causes** – the functions, which disturbed, leads to the illness.

In X's case, this would refer to the blockage of the coronary artery brought about by the formation of a blood clot, and it's lodging in a particularly narrow section of one of the heart's blood vessels. This would be the manifestation of the causes – a consequence of the final outcome associated with a function of the body.

Persian Medicine identifies two basic origins of clinical disorders:

1. **Internal origin** – these are diseases that originate within the body due to a humoral, temperamental (qualitative) or functional imbalance.

(For example, inflammation of the gastric mucosa can lead to gastric ulcers.)

2. **External origin** – those arising from outside the body.

(For example, an injury leading to pain or an ailment arises from poor diet, bad weather, lack of exercise, invasion by microbes and emotional stimuli.)

The sequence of cause and effect, externally and internally

An example of external causes influencing health which has been supplied by Ibn Sina is as follows.

If a person consumes hot and dry foods to excess, and other related external hot and dry causes, such as hot weather and anger, are present, an imbalance in the bilious humor can occur. This imbalance originating externally can then become the cause for the internal conditions of inflammation of the liver – hepatitis – which can result in the symptoms of nausea, vomiting, shivering, jaundice and fever.

Effects on the body resulting from different causes

Ibn Sina listed a number of internal and external factors which can cause different forms of structural or functional disorders which themselves can lead on to specific symptoms of bodily disorders.

- Increase in body temperature – can result from putrefaction (infection), or from excessive consumption of hot foods or drinks.

- Decrease in body temperature – can result from excessive sleep, overeating cold and moist foods, constipation, and certain drugs (humectants).

- Excessive dryness – results from over-exercise, wakefulness, intercourse, desiccant drugs (diuretics), and starvation.

- Blockage of vessels – results from growths (tumours), kidney stones, blockage (embolism).

- Dyspepsia – results from lack of exercise, overeating, lack of depletion (slow stomach emptying).

- Channels dilating – results from constipation, diarrhea.

- Excessive skin smoothness or roughness – results from the application of caustic solutions, detergents, acids, solvents and plaster.

- Ulceration – results from the rupture of skin blisters, sepsis, corrosive pustules, and local acidic environment.

Other points made by Ibn Sina:

(a) The effect of a particular cause may change from person to person. It may have a different response in strong or weak persons, or in sensitive or insensitive individuals. This is another example supporting the uniqueness of the individual.

(b) The same cause may give rise to different diseases in different people. For example, high blood pressure in one person may lead to kidney failure, in another person to a stroke, and in a third person to heart failure.

Causes of disease associated with temperament

Each person has a unique temperament that is ideal, or optimum, for him or her.

Temperament and pre-disposition towards disease – formal cause

It is important to know the person's particular temperament, as it provides vital clues as to which disorders he or she will be susceptible to. The temperament will reflect a number of influences – the genetic make-up, the physical, organic constraints operating on him or her.

Information from the research project gathered over the years has substantiated this relationship of temperament and pre-disposition towards illness conditions.

However, the relationship between temperament and health (or disease) is based on the change in the ideal qualitative state of the person in relation to his/ her temperament. When a person's optimum qualitative state is disturbed, then a trend towards disease begins. If this trend is not corrected by the person's physis, then the signs and symptoms of a particular disorder will appear.

Person with a dominant sanguineous temperament (Hot & Moist) plus sub-dominant phlegmatic temperament (Cold & Moist) will have an ideal qualitative state that has a highest level of moistness, followed by heat, then coldness, and then the least amount of dryness.

This ideal qualitative state associated with a person's temperament will invariably bestow on this person a predisposition to certain states of health or disease.

Changes to this ideal qualitative state will have a negative influence on the person's health.

Temperament and the environment

Changes to the person's ideal qualitative state can only take place during the interaction between an individual and the environment. This highlights the fact that even though temperament can have predispositions to states of health and disease, it is ulimately the interaction between an individual (microcosm), and the environment (macrocosm) that will be the cause of disease.

Whilst temperament is considered to be the cause of health and disease, it is ulimately dependent on the lifestyle factors.

Causes associated with Humors

Causes associated with humors – *material causes* – can happen (a) qualitatively from the effects of heat, coldness, dryness and moistness, and/or (b) quantitatively, resulting from different concentrations of the four humors.

Humors are produced in the liver from the food and drink we consume. One of the most important functions of the humors is to maintain the person's ideal qualitative state, so that it is in harmony with his or her qualitative requirements.

Humoral changes resulting from food and drink

If a person consumes food and drink which is improper or unsuitable, an excess of a particular humor will be produced which is not ideally suited to the person.

For example, if a person with a dominant bilious (Hot & Dry) temperament eats excessively hot & dry foods, this will lead to the formation of too much bilious humor. As a result, the ideal composition of humors required for the person will change, specifically increasing the amount of the qualities of heat and dryness above the ideal for this person.

Similarly, if the same person eats too much in the way of cold & moist foods, the excessive phlegmatic humor which will follow will again change the ideal composition of humors. This will reduce the ideal hot & dry qualities associated with the person's bilious temperament.

These changes in humors therefore affect the person:

(a) Quantitatively – by increasing or decreasing the amounts of the different humors

(b) Qualitatively – by affecting the relative composition or ratio of the different humors

Either way, an imbalance develops in the person's ideal humoral and temperamental nature.

Humoral changes resulting from lifestyle factors

A person may have the ideal, optimum balance of humors, both quantitatively and qualitatively, because he or she eats and drinks sensibly and avoids excess, but changes can occur to ideal the combination of humors because of other lifestyle factors.

For example, if a person reacts badly to stress or fails to achieve good sleep hygiene, the resultant negative impact will alter the person's ideal qualitative state of the humors, as required by the temperament. This imbalance in humors will inevitably lead to a situation favouring the development of illness.

Causes associated with Function

The body's structure is continually being regenerated by means of cell division and a whole range of metabolic activities. The body fluids and humors are the agents for this regeneration. Humors also maintain the temperament of the structure that has been produced. Food and drink provide the body fluids with the essential materials for the regeneration of cells.

The maintenance of both temperament of organs/tissues as well as the structure to perform efficient functions is dependent on the humors of the body.

As the ideal humoral balance of an individual is dependent on lifestyle factors, especially diet, causes associated with functions *(final cause)* are also dependent on the lifestyle factors.

This is in keeping with the philosophy:

"All living organisms grow at the expense of the environment, taking from it what is necessary and rejecting what is unnecessary." [Hippocrates]

It is the effective digestion of the environment that constitutes health. However, if poorly managed it becomes the cause of disease.

Causes associated with the Lifestyle Factors

The individual's environment is identified in terms of the Lifestyle factors.

♦ The lifestyle factors are ulimately responsible for the development of disease and the maintenance of health

Six of these are common to all individuals.

- Environmental air and breathing

- Food and drink

- Movement and rest

- Our emotional life

- Sleep and wakefulness

• Elimination and retention

There are other factors which have varying influences in specific circumstances.

• Occupation or career

• Place of residence

• Exposure to toxic substances

• Exposure to pathogenic organisms

• Age, gender

• Personal habits

The Lifestyle factors, especially the six major ones, influence each and every one of us in keeping with the philosophy of Persian Medicine.

Persian Medicine considers that disturbances in these Lifestyle factors are the primary causes of all illnesses. *(Efficient cause)*

Environmental Air and Breathing

The air we breathe is the most important living connection with our environment – from the moment we are born, to the time of our death.

The air we breathe is the first step in the hierarchy of physiological needs. Its role in the maintenance of health is too often neglected or ignored completely

"Air is the author of life, disease and death to the people" *[Culpeper]*

Air is the main thing that all living organisms share on Earth. It flows between us all, connecting us intimately.

Physis is actively involved in maintaining the balance between the body's need for oxygen, and its need to remove toxins from the body.

The function of air in health and disease

Air is composed of mainly nitrogen (around 74%), oxygen (25%) and carbon dioxide (0.5%, and rising), plus a number of rare gases such as helium, methane and argon. The oxygen in environmental air is the only component used by human beings.

The air we inhale and exhale has several vital functions:

• Air is our primary source of nutrition. The oxygen contained in air is needed to transform the nutrients present in our food into energy and into the humors and body fluids that maintain the body.

• Air also diminishes excessive heat, so helping maintain our ideal body temperature.

• Air cleanses the body of some forms of waste matter, like carbon dioxide and volatile gases formed in the breakdown of, for example, garlic in the food.

"Air is the fountain of life, and also provides the source for the activation of energies to form humors and body fluids and maintain life" [Hippocrates].

There is a growing body of evidence suggesting that changes in temperature, humidity, air speed and pollution can lead to increases in the number of people who have heart attacks, strokes, respiratory problems and other disorders. Persian Medicine has long recognised this.

Climates do influence diseases. In recognition of this, some medical schools have separate departments of tropical medicine, recognising that heat and humidity in the air that we breathe can make the person more vulnerable to certain diseases. In Iran we are aware that people living in different regions are more prone to certain diseases. Intestinal complaints are more prevalent in Hot climates, chest diseases in cold, moist climates, and skin disorders in moist and hot climates.

Purity of air

We require clean, healthy air to breathe, and maintain our optimum health.

By far the most important aspect of health is the nature and severity of pollution in the atmosphere. Industrial smoke is now accepted as the worst offender, and a real danger to life. However, domestic pollution – from cooking or heating fires – is also a serious problem. The air we breathe should be neither contaminated by industrial pollutants, domestic activity or car exhaust fumes, made stale by people who are confined to homes, offices, airliners and social venues without proper ventilation.

If the quality of air is poor, then the onset and development of specific diseases can be accelerated. In fact, many occupational diseases have their origin in lungs weakened by exposure to poor quality air.

Examples of diseases related to the quality of environmental air

• Bronchitis. There is no doubt that this disease is linked to pollution in a cold and damp climate – hence the nickname 'the English disease'.

• Bronchial asthma (allergic) this disorder is on the increase in areas where diesel fumes and other air-borne toxins are becoming concentrated.

• Fibrosis of the lung. This can arise from dust and smoke in the air breathed by industrial workers over a long period of time

• Asbestosis. This life-threatening disorder often afflicts miners working in asbestos mines

• Cancer. Small metallic particles in the air are linked to lung cancer.

• Stroke. Air pollution increases the risk of having a stroke

Today, environmental factors of all sorts, especially air pollutants, are being implicated in the development of several diseases.

Air as a carrier of infectious disease

We are all familiar with the fact that the different seasons of the year bring with them different diseases.

Persian Medicine physicians were unable to identify micro-organisms (viruses, bacteria and fungi) because at the time they lacked the appropriate technology. However, they recognised that different seasons bring with them different illnesses. These illnesses are the result of the changes of qualities in the air which allows for greater multiplication of certain bacteria and other micro-organisms under conditions which are ideal for this.

This explains why certain ailments are more prevalent at different times of the year. For example, viral respiratory infections are more prevalent in winter (coryza and influenza), respiratory allergic disorders (hay fever) in spring, and several gastro-intestinal problems, measles, chicken pox and fungal infections in summer.

The relationship between air as a carrier of infectious diseases can easily be explained according to Ibn Sina's conditions necessary for a cause to have an effect. As mentioned earlier, the following three conditions are necessary:

Active power: Using *the* winter season example quoted above; there may be sufficient active power. The person may be exposed to a highly pathogenic viral or bacterial load in the air that is breathed. Also, the person may be exposed to a particular microbe or toxin for the very first time, so will react very definitely.

(1) **Receptive power**. Because of the person's favourable internal environment, the microbes will only be capable of exerting a pathological impact if there is sufficient receptive power within the individual's humor, or if the individual's immune system is compromised. This is more likely to happen if the person has not come into earlier contact with the pathogen or toxin. Also certain temperamental types will be more inclined than others to certain illness conditions.

(2) **Prolonged contact**. The third condition relates to the need for prolonged contact between the micro-organism and the person. This means that even if a person's humoral balance is strong enough initially to withstand the onslaught of the bacteria or virus, over a sustained period the immune system can become compromised. This is more likely to happen in conditions of overcrowding, or in institutions such as schools and prisons, where people are in very close proximity to each other.

Temperamental quality of environmental air and its effects

Environmental air interacts significantly with the person's temperament.

Generally, the quality of air may contribute to the development of ill-health in a person. This is a factor which should be considered when job relocating, retiring or emigrating – the person should be aware of the benefits and drawbacks arising from the environmental air he or she will be breathing. A number of situations are shown below.

Qualities of atmospheric air which can affect health

a) Atmospheric wind – hot or cold, moist or dry, direction, high or low velocity

b) The domestic situation – room temperature, cooking odours, paint fumes, circulating fresh or stale air

c) The local terrain – coastal or inland, sheltered or exposed, or high or low elevation

d) Pollutants – both visible (soot particles) and invisible (carbon monoxide and sulphur dioxide)

e) The presence of ionised particles – such a positive or negative ions, free radicals, or radioactive decay products like argon

f) In terms of temperament, air is considered Hot & Moist, but can vary from region to region, due to its geographical size and variety of eco-systems. For example, in the coastal regions it is Hot & Moist, being more humid, and on the inland plateau it is more Cold & Dry. These differences will have different effects on different people.

Recent information on the effect of air quality on health

There is increasing evidence that changes in temperature, humidity, air speed, and pollution can lead to highly predictable increases in the number of people who have strokes, heat attacks, and respiratory disorders.

Air pollution

♦ This can prove fatal. It poses a greater threat to health, causing more early deaths than previously believed. Not only does it affect overall mortality, but increases the incidence of ischemic heart disease, asthma and lung cancer.

♦ Thunderstorms have been linked to a higher incidence of hay fever, due to the circulation by the disturbed air of pollen and spores and toxins.

♦ The use of burning mosquito coils is harmful to children especially, as hey are known to produce very toxic by-products.

Workplace toxins

♦ Skin reactions, asthma and ear disorders due to the person's workplace, especially the floor, chair, desk and computer, being contaminated by toxins which readily circulate in the air encouraged by electrostatic charges. The toxins include fragments of insects, particularly cockroaches and mites, plant pollen. In fact, offices are more toxic than public toilets.

♦Occupational and domestic exposure to paint fumes should always be avoided as they are toxic and associated with several negative health effects, such as headaches and nausea.

Cigarette smoking

♦The deleterious effects of 'side stream' cigarette smoke have been suspected for some time. Now there is considerable evidence that the dangers to innocent bystanders are real and substantial. Not only watery eyes, asthma attacks in the short term, but bronchitis, skin disorders and various cancers in the longer period.

♦Since the no smoking rule was introduced, the improvement in people's health is definitely noticeable.

Hot and cold weather

♦Heat waves, when the air temperature is excessive both day and night, lead to heat exhaustion, heat strokes, heart attacks and strokes.

♦Low temperatures stress the body. Heart attacks increase after bitter cold weather. Deaths from respiratory disorders also increase after a cold snap.

Environmental air and the individual

People are affected differently by air, depending on their individual temperament.

Unfortunately, a person cannot control the weather. However, by knowing the temperament of the patient, you could advise him or her to compensate for adverse weather conditions by maintaining their ideal temperamental quality by actively invoking other lifestyle factors, especially diet and exercise.

People with different temperaments will be affected differently by certain weather scenarios. A number of these are shown below.

Temperament and response to weather conditions

- Persons with a dominant sanguineous temperament will be most affected by the overall heat of summer, especially on the coast

- Persons with a dominant phlegmatic temperament will be most affected by the overall coldness of winter, especially on the coast

- Persons with a dominant bilious temperament will be most affected by the overall heat of summer, especially in dry regions

- Persons with a dominant melancholic temperament will be most affected by the overall coldness of winter, especially in dry regions

Air conditioners

As air conditioners are a central feature of daily life in the world, it is important to be aware that they can be a serious health hazard, especially in confined spaces like airliners, hospitals, teaching establishments and offices.

Many illnesses are the result of exposure to air conditioners, which are known to be very effective in rapidly spreading disease-causing microbes, toxins and allergens. These are responsible for sudden qualitative changes which can arise from their use. Persons suffering from sinus problems or bronchial asthma are hardly likely to recover completely from these illnesses, no matter what treatment they are receiving, if the air conditioner is a contributory cause.

Most air conditioners increase the qualities of coldness and dryness of the immediate environment. Therefore, those people most likely to be adversely affected would be people with a phlegmatic or melancholic temperament. In addition, other temperamental types could conceivably be affected by the sudden changes from hot to cold to hot, etc. Even persons with dominant sanguineous and bilious temperaments will be affected negatively.

Breathing techniques

The manner in which we breathe can affect our health, even when the quality of the air is fine.

Poor breathing habits are a major underlying cause of a number of illnesses. Often symptoms like headaches, fatigue and irritability arise from poor, inefficient breathing, which results in low, sub-optimal levels of circulating oxygen in the body.

A correct breathing technique can overcome strong emotions like anger and fear. It may also help in reduce the symptoms of anxiety – trembling, palpitations, sweating – which arise, for example, in interviews, public speaking and competitions.

Food and drink

For practitioners of Persian Medicine, food is seen as the major external factor in the maintenance of health, and the chief medicine at their disposal.

“Leave your drugs in the chemist’s pot if you can heal the patient with food” [Hippocrates]

Also:

‘All diseases begin at the stomach” *[Prophet Mohammed (PBUH)]*

There is more and more data linking the food we consume to different diseases.

The world is facing an accelerating pandemic of obesity. Being obese doubles your chance of getting bowel and breast cancer and causes osteoarthritis, diabetes, hypertension and lung disease. And excessive eating raises levels of cholesterol, which accumulates in your arteries causing strokes and heart attacks. Socially, too, obesity is a disaster. People who are overweight are depressed, they have a lower than average income, a higher divorce rate and commit suicide more often. Obesity is probably the single most important reason why, in spite of all the advances in medicine and sanitation, we are not living much longer than people a 100 years ago.

Whereas some lifestyle factors, such as the air we breathe and our emotional state, cannot be rigorously controlled, a certain amount of choice exists with other lifestyle factors, such as our sleeping patterns and exercise and rest. However, the food and drink we consume is the one lifestyle factor over which we have absolute control, as the process is purely voluntary. People can be empowered in their decision regarding what enters, or not enters, their stomach.

Food is the raw material the body uses for the production of the four humors. Therefore, the quality and quantity of the food consumed has a direct impact on the quality and quantity of the humors produced by the body.

Food can be classified in different ways. Some are shown below:

Classification of foods

- Conventionally – divided chemically into proteins, fats, carbohydrates and minerals

- Nutrition-wise – allocated to groups which provide nutrition and energy, either in different densities or at different rates

- Protection-wise –- foods which can boost the immune system or contain anti-oxidants

• Value-wise – food which are 'good' for you (health foods) and those which are 'bad' for you (junk foods)

In Persian Medicine, a particular food is classified according to the temperament of its nutritional components into either heating or cooling, with appropriate levels of moisture or dryness.

The concept of heating and cooling applied to foods is linked to the effect of the foods on the body. Foods which are heating in nature will increase the rate of metabolism. Conversely, foods which are cooling in nature will reduce the body's metabolic rate.

It is evidenced that all foods – meat, vegetables, grains, etc. – have qualities associated with them. If we add the concept of qualities to the standard classification and then we can see the relationship between proteins, fats, carbohydrates, minerals and qualities.

• Protein – Overall quality of Dryness, but with degrees of heat or coldness, and the least amount of moistness

• Fats – Overall quality of Heat, but with degrees of moistness, and the least amount of dryness and coldness

• Carbohydrates – Overall quality of Moistness, but with degrees of heat and coldness, and the least amount of dryness

• Water – Overall quality of Cold and Moistness.

• Minerals – Overall quality of Cold and Dryness.

The biochemistry of the body depends not only on the quantity of food we eat but also on the quality of the food we take in.

When providing dietary advice for a patient, the practitioner should ask three questions:

1. What will produce or restore the balance in the four humors?

2. What is the particular temperament of the individual?

3. What is appropriate for his or her age, the season of the year, and the climate in which he or she lives?

A balanced diet which includes heating and cooling foods is absolutely essential for the maintenance of good health.

A diet in which nutrients consumed in excess of the body's needs or its ability to digest it will produce an imbalance of humors. Also, the undigested food can lead to plethora, a feeling of fullness or satiety, in which food accumulates without elimination.

Food and the maintenance of body heat

Correct body heat is necessary so that metabolism in general and enzyme activity in particular can proceed effectively. A confirmation of Persian Medicine's view of the metabolic efficiency of foods and digestion is found in recent research on enzymes. Research reveals that when spices such as ginger, cumin and cinnamon – the heating spices – are consumed, the production of digestive enzymes by the body increases dramatically, so facilitating digestion and improving elimination. (Edward Howell)

According to Persian Medicine, 'heating' foods and spices:

• Increase the production of digestive enzymes in the gastro-intestinal tract.

• Increase the efficiency of functioning at the cellular and metabolic levels.

• Facilitates the assimilation of micronutrients, with a minimum of metabolic waste.

• Achieve and maintain complete metabolic digestion.

The typical western diet, which relies heavily on meat (overall dryness), pastas and salads (overall cold), etc. would invariably increase the cold and dry qualities within the body. This is opposite to the maintenance of the body's ideal temperament, which is hot (normal temperature 37ºC) and moist (contains 60% to 70% moisture). Not unexpectedly, "diseases of lifestyle" such as diabetes, obesity, atherosclerosis and rheumatic disorders are positively encouraged to develop by long term adherence to the typical Western diet.

According to Persian Medicine, many serious diseases arise from an excess of cold and dry temperament, aggravated by a lack of body heat.

Many articles are available on the benefits of Asian cuisine which includes the use of ginger, garlic and other heating herbs and spices.

Temperamental Qualities of Tastes

Persian Medicine has also linked qualities with the taste of foods.

Taste	**Qualities**
Salty	Hot and dry
Sweet	Moist and Hot
Sour	Cold and Dry
Bitter	Dry and Hot
Pungent or spicy	Hot and Dry
Tasteless or bland	Cold and moist

The Effects of taste and qualities on individuals

• **Salty or tangy taste** - Hot and dry foods

Excessive intake of salty foods increases the Heat and dryness qualities.

These commonly consumed foods – for example, many snack foods – can be harmful to the heart, increase the blood pressure, and can lead to electrolyte imbalance, congestive headache, dizziness, vertigo, stroke or paralysis of the right side. They may also confer a greenish tinge on the complexion.

Examples: common salt, salty foods

The qualitative effects of salty foods are counteracted by foods having are tasteless (cold and moist).

• **Sweet taste** - Moist and Hot foods

Eating sweet foods to excess will increase the Moistness and Heat qualities of the body.

These foods can be harmful to the spleen, pancreas and kidneys. They can also favor the onset of diabetes, sluggish spleen and arthritis.

Examples: cakes, biscuits, sweetmeats

The qualitative effects of sweet foods are counteracted by foods having a sour and astringent taste (cold and dry).

• **No taste or insipid taste** - Cold and Moist foods

Excess of insipid foods increases the Coldness and Moistness qualities of the body.

These foods are potentially harmful to the glands, metabolism and vital faculties. They also decrease the hemoglobin level, so promoting anemia. In addition, they can lead to hypothyroidism, amenorrhea, and anorexia, high level of lipids (dyslipidemia), sluggish liver, impotence and loss of hair.

Examples: cucumber, radish, fruits containing lots of water, such as watermelon

The qualitative effects of insipid foods are counteracted by foods having a bitter, acid or tart taste (dry and hot).

• Sour taste - Cold and Dry foods

Excessive consumption of sour and astringent food increases the Cold and Dry qualities.

This can negatively affect the digestive and nervous systems, and encourages thicker blood in the circulatory system. The net effect can be illnesses such as hyperacidity, weakness of the nerves (neuritis), thrombosis, arteriosclerosis, constipation, kidney stones, psoriasis and gout. The skin is more likely to become dry and wrinkled.

Examples: sour fruits such as lemon, grapefruit, etc., fish (astringent)

The qualitative effects of sour and astringent foods (cold & dry) are counteracted or overcome by foods having a pungent, spicy or seasoned taste (hot and dry).

• Bitter taste - Dry and Hot foods

An excessive intake of bitter foods increases the Dry and Hot qualities in the body.

They can be harmful to the lungs and the arteries, and may promote excessive bleeding. The net effect may be provocation of illnesses such as tuberculosis and bleeding piles. They also tend to dry out the skin.

Examples: bitter gourd, fenugreek seeds, nutmeg, cinnamon, cloves

The qualitative effects of bitter foods are counteracted by foods having a salty or tangy taste (hot and moist).

• Pungent or spicy taste - Hot and Dry foods

Pungent foods taken in abnormally large portions increase the Heat and Dryness qualities.

Foods flavored according to this taste are potentially harmful to the liver, and can weaken the heart's muscular tone. The net effect may be conditions such as jaundice, hepatitis and cardiomegaly (enlargement of the heart).

Examples: red chilies, garlic

The qualitative effects of pungent foods are counteracted by foods having a sweet or honeyed taste (moist and hot).

The effects of qualities on specific temperaments

The above effects of taste on individuals will be increased or enhanced if the tastes and the quality associated with it are similar to the individual's dominant temperamental quality. For example, an individual who is dominant Bilious (Hot & Dry) will be affected much more by foods with pungent, spicy or seasoned foods (which are Hot & Dry) or bitter, acid or tart foods (which are Dry & Hot)

Mixing foods with different qualities

Current ideas in therapeutic dieting advocate that proteins and carbohydrates should not be mixed in the same serving. Persian Medicine has ly discouraged the consuming of many dishes and tastes at the same meal. For example, milk products should not be eaten at the same time as sour foodstuffs. The combination of milk products with sour things in the same meal would interfere with the digestive process, and cause flatulence and bloating. Also, fish should not be taken at the same time as milk or milkshakes. Indeed, milk (as a large portion) should be avoided at any meal.

Temperature of foods

Whilst specific foods may have their own inherent qualities, the temperature at which the foods and drinks are consumed can also have negative effects. Bearing in mind that the average body temperature is 37°C, consuming foods at temperatures close to the body's temperature will have the least amount of negative effect. The common practice of ice drinks, especially in winter, is an aggravating factor for many disorders.

Water

One of the most important needs of the body is water, in order to maintain the body's 70% moisture content. Water plays an important role in the processes of food digestion, nutrient metabolism, and elimination of waste products. It also ensures the proper circulation of blood and lymph. Virtually every function of the body, from cell division to food digestion to tissue synthesis requires adequate moisture levels. The importance of the maintenance of the ideal moisture content is therefore self-evident.

The human body is capable of dealing with an excessive water intake. However, it is unable to handle an inadequate water intake. Many illnesses result from inadequate water intake. For example, kidney stones and kidney failure result from dehydration. An adequate intake of water helps in reducing raised blood pressure, elevated levels of cholesterol, uric acid and glucose in the body.

Movement and rest

A balance between physical activity, or movement, and relaxation, or rest, is essential for the maintenance of good health.

The concept of exercise can have important implications when viewed from the perspective of Persian Medicine. Movement and rest have an effect on the overall heat and moistness that is associated with the temperament of the human body with the appropriate variations of the individual temperament. Therefore, excess of either movement or rest will have harmful effects.

Movement and exercise

Energy must be expended for movement to occur, and the result of movement is the production of body heat.

People vary enormously in the relative proportion of time and effort they allocate either to physical exercise, or to relaxation. Some people can endure greater degrees of physical activity or movement; others need more rest and relaxation. This wide variation between movement and rest is determined by the temperament of the individual.

Initially, movement (or exercise) produces levels of heat dependent on the extent and intensity of the physical activity. This increased level of heat will result in a decrease of moisture, and an increase in dryness.

As the physical activity continues, a state of diminished heat and moistness will come about, which then progresses into a state of coldness and dryness.

This could result in an overall loss of body functions.

Persons who are endowed with extra heat and moistness (such as the sanguineous temperament) will be less affected as compared to a person whose temperament has a quality of dryness and coldness associated with it (such as the bilious temperament).

Adequate and appropriate movement (exercise) is necessary to maintain an ideal body temperament of an individual. The wrong choice of exercise or excessive movement is the cause of many illnesses.

For example, a couple join a health club. They both participate in a spinning exercise (excessive cycling at a heavy pace, for at least 45 minutes). The husband (dominant sanguineous – Hot & Moist; subdominant phlegmatic – Cold & Moist) had no negative effects as his temperament had adequate moisture to balance the increase heat level. On the other hand his wife (dominant melancholic – Cold & Dry; subdominant bilious – Hot & Dry) developed an overactive thyroid gland due to an increase in heat & dryness from the exercise.

Physical rest

Life is a constant flux between movement and rest.

This is highlighted by the periods of rest between the heart beats, breathing, and in fact all functions of the body are governed by this constant interchange between movement and rest. Lack of good quality rest has a disturbing effect on a person's physis, making him or her more susceptible to illnesses.

However just as too much movement is possibly harmful, excessive rest is not good for the body. Resting increases moisture in the body. If this becomes excessive, this will cool the body down, and eventually lead the body towards becoming cold and moist. Finally, an excessively cold and dry condition will develop. This could also progress to overall loss of body functions.

Unfortunately, many people are unable to rest properly because:

(a) they are over-stimulationd by the caffeine present in tea, coffee and coke;

(b) they are affected by stimulant drugs often present in cold and flu preparations, or herbal mixtures containing ephedrine, for example;

(c) their environment is too noisy or distracting;

(d) They are suffering from miscellaneous aches and pains.

It is interesting to note that excess of movement (exercise) will have the same final result as rest in terms of qualities of Cold and dry, so affecting bodily functions similarly.

Some proven health benefits of exercise

♦The heart: Regular, mild to moderate exercise is good for the heart

♦The brain: Exercise helps to protect against stroke in those people who are at risk

♦Excess body mass: Regular helps to reduce excessive body mass, and to keep it that way

♦Bone mass: Together with good nutrition, regular, low-impact exercise prevents osteoporosis

♦Blood pressure: Exercise is good for maintaining normal blood pressure

♦Stress: Exercise helps reduce the impact of constant mental or emotional stress

♦Colds and flu: People who exercise are less likely to get respiratory infections

♦Asthma: The severity of asthmatic attacks is less in those who exercise regularly

♦Diabetes: The complications of diabetes are minimised in people who exercise

♦Sleep: Relaxation exercise help in insomnia – and for recurrent headache and backache

♦Impotence: Exercise helps to combat sexual problems, especially impotence

♦Mental, emotional health: Regular, reasonable exercise helps to maintain good mental and emotional health status

Our Emotions

Emotions are known to play a major role in the maintenance of health.

Naturalists strongly emphasize the importance of how the mind can play a significant role in the healing process.

Research has revealed time and time again the value and benefit of positive attitude on the maintenance of health, and in assisting the processes of healing and recovery. Of interest is that the relatively new healing discipline, psycho-neuro-immunology (PNI) is based on the premise that the conscious mind (psycho), the central nervous system (neuro) and the body's defences (immuno) are interconnected, and combine and actively co-operate in the healing process.

A good example of how emotions can affect an individual's health emerges from clinical trials in which placebos (so-called inactive drug forms) are compared to active conventional drugs. Very often the participants receiving the placebos exhibit the same or very similar quantitative improvement as do the participants who are receiving the active drug.

According to Persian Medicine, excessive, uncontrolled emotion may be functionally damaging. The mind can play a significant role in helping the healing process, and a positive attitude can play a major part in the prognosis of a particular illness.

An inclination towards certain emotions is inherent in an individual's personality. This is part of a person's genetic make-up. People respond differently under similar circumstances. Whilst some people can handle stress, others cannot. Some people by nature are calm, others are easily ruffled. Reaction to a particular environment or situation results in emotional states that can seriously affect a person's health. Emotions such as anger produces heat, which leads to palpitations, and fear leads to disturbances in moistness, which leads to sweaty palms.

The influence of emotions manifests itself by the temperamental qualities associated with emotions. Listed below are the qualitative effects of different emotions:

Anger	Hot and Dry
Worry	Hot and Moist
Depression	Moist and Hot
Fear	Cold and Moist
Grief	Cold and Dry
Excitement	Dry and Hot

Ibn Sina was one of the pioneers who wrote extensively on the effects of suppressed or uncontrolled emotions. Persian Medicine over the centuries has recognized the effect, and the relationship between emotions and specific illnesses. The effect of the respective emotion is linked to the quality associated with the individual as well as the quality associated with the emotion. For example, if a bilious person whose temperament is Hot & Dry is influenced by anger, which has the similar quality of Hot & Dry, the negative effect of anger in this individual will be intensified.

Listed below are the negative effects of the qualities of respective emotions:

- Anger (Hot & Dry quality)

Excessive anger can be harmful to the liver, and also badly affect the digestive process. Anger produces Stimulation in the liver. In anger the blood circulation suddenly diverts to the skin. With this emotion a lot of heat is produced in the body, which can harm the internal organs. This requires Physis to shift the circulation outward in order to protect the internal organs from damage. Episodes of anger produce harmful effects in the heart, and liver, damages the brain. Anger is associated with the bilious temperament, and increases the bilious humor.

• Worries (Hot & Moist quality)

Excessive worries can cause disease of the pancreas, resulting in an imbalance of glucose levels.

• Depression (Moist & Hot quality)

Excessive depression is harmful to the brain and weakens all faculties. Depression stimulates the phlegmatic humor.

• Fear (Cold & Moist quality)

Excessive fear leads to diseases of the kidneys and bladder, and weakens the adrenal and posterior pituitary glands. In fear the blood circulation suddenly moves inwards, resulting in the face and skin becoming pale and cold, and breathing becoming shallow. Because of this emotion a lot of cold develops in the body, so Physis shifts the circulation inwards to protect the internal organs from damage. Fear also produces negative effects in the liver and heart.

• Grief (Cold & Dry quality)

Excessive grief is an acute condition of the nervous system. It weakens the nerve impulses and produces negative effects on the brain, lungs, heart and liver.

• Excitement (Dry & Hot quality)

Excessive excitement can be harmful to the heart. Circulation gradually surfaces to the skin; the face and skin become red and hot, and breathing increases. With excitement a lot of heat is produced in the body, which can harm the internal organs, Physis shifts the circulation outward to protect the internal organs from this damage.

From the above descriptions, it can be observed that emotions (with their respective qualities) play a crucial role in an individual's well-being.

It is extremely important to recognise and search for the effect of emotions as being the cause of many illnesses. The health professional needs to be aware of this and should always include this factor in the treatment programme.

"Some patients, though their condition is perilous, recover their health simply through their contentment with the goodness of the physician." *[Hippocrates]*

Sleep and wakefulness

According to Persian Medicine, sleep is seen as cooling and moistening. It affords Physis the opportunity for uninterrupted action in restoring the body's harmonies. Wakefulness increases dryness and heat and depletes energies from physical and mental activity.

Sleep renews and maintains physical and psychological performance. Sleep strengthens all natural functions, including digestion, metabolism, and brain power. During sleep the body restores itself from fatigue and gives Physis the opportunity to prepare for the elimination of toxins and the opportunity to focus on repair and restoration of health.

When a person perspires heavily during sleep without any obvious cause, it means that undigested and unwanted fluids have accumulated in excess of the bodily requirements. With the help of sleep these unwanted matters are eliminated through the skin.

Sleep strengthens all natural functions, including:

(a) Digestive processes, which it helps to complete, ready for bowel movement on awakening;

(b) Metabolic processes, which repairs damage and restores integrity, primarily under the influence of the parasympathetic nervous system;

(c) Brain functions, by sorting out and filing sensory and intellectual input from the previous day.

(d) Detoxification, by assisting physis in eliminating toxins from the system.

The requirement for sleep differs from person to person, and also for different age groups. The amount of sleep needed will also be influenced by the extent of physical or mental activity which the person undergoes through the day. Generally, women need more sleep than do men, and children more than adults. Also, the elderly will benefit from extra sleep, as the moisture will overcome the dryness associated with old age.

Sleep requirements vary widely, according to temperament:

- Persons with a dominant bilious temperament – 5 to 6 hours minimum nightly;

- Persons with a dominant melancholic temperament – 5 to 6 hours minimum nightly;

- Persons with a sanguineous temperament – 6 to 7 hours minimum nightly;

- Persons with a dominant phlegmatic temperament – at least 8 hours nightly.

Insufficient sleep leads to excessive heat and dryness affecting all individuals especially a person with a bilious temperament. This condition can be easily reversed with an appropriate amount of sleep that will help reduce the excess heat and dryness as sleep has a cooling and moistening effect on the body.

Insomnia is quite a prevalent problem especially amongst the individuals with a Cold & Dry (melancholic) qualitative state. Excessive dryness is the cause behind insomnia (which is why very often a glass of Hot milk, which is hot & moist in temperament, seems to help). Obviously if a person does not get enough sleep, it will affect the person's mental, physical and emotional states. Troubled sleep indicates that a disease may be developing, Excessive awakening brings about conditions of headaches, slurred speech, lack of concentration, mood swings, irritability, lethargy, melancholia, etc.

Today's lifestyle (entertainment, TV, etc.) invariably leads to a chronic sleep debt, which often results in serious consequences.

Excessive rest and sleep (hypersomnia) gives rise to an excessiveness of a Cold & Moist temperament which is harmful for the vital, metabolic and psychic faculties affecting the level of available energy. Long periods of increased Cold & Moistness increase the weakness of the muscles, disturb the digestion and metabolism, and dull the mind, increased phlegm in the body, bradycardia, weak memory and low blood pressure, etc.

Elimination and Retention

Waste products are substances which are of no further use to the body.

According to Persian Medicine, the relationship between an individual and the environment is a dynamic process of consuming and retaining what is necessary to support life, and efficiently eliminating the waste that has accumulated. Persian Medicine subscribes to the philosophy that the stomach is the home of all illnesses.

Retention within the body

The term 'retention' is linked to the metabolic faculty (under control of the liver) to ensure that nutrients are retained long enough for the assimilation to be effective and then eliminated. Very often a person may consume nutritious food but the body is unable to assimilate the nutrients. Improper functioning in the metabolic faculty will inhibit effective metabolism and the ideal period of retention will not be met thus having negative effects on the body.

Accumulation of toxins interferes with normal biochemical processes of the body.

This impairs not only basic bodily functions, but also affect the further continuous processing of food and drink into ideal humors. This would then introduce more toxins into the system and eventually overcome the ability of physis to maintain health. The presence of toxins places great burdens on the liver, kidney and the lungs eventually causing serious damage to these important organs.

The body has many levels of dealing with abnormal physiological functions, from built-in repair and screening mechanisms, to sophisticated levels of interception by the immune system. Invariably toxins or abnormal humors which invade the bloodstream or tissues can cause illnesses associated with tissue, organ damage and even cancers.

As mentioned before the human body is a very complex system completely integrated and interdependent. Whilst a person may be suffering from a headache or mouth sores and the link between this and a toxin-filled colon may not be apparent, but in Persian Medicine this link as the cause is clearly identified.

"The effective digestion, assimilation and elimination of the lifestyle factors constitute health."

Retention also applies to the inefficiency of the body to eliminate wastes, as is the case with ascites.

Elimination from the body

As these waste products are toxic if they accumulate excessively in the body, they must be expelled regularly and totally.

Elimination is a term which embraces all natural functions in which waste products are removed from the body.

There are four main routes of excretion:

- Via the kidney – by urination, as urine;
- Via the feces – by defecation, as feces (stool);
- Via the lung – by respiration, as volatile substances;
- Via the skin – by perspiration, as visible or invisible sweating.

These are the main excretory systems. However, there are a number of others which also contribute to toxic waste expulsion. These include coughing, sneezing, nasal mucus, vomiting, flatulence, menstruation, ear wax and ejaculation.

Elimination can only be efficient if and when all the metabolic functions are in order. If the Lifestyle factors are well managed and functions are normal, elimination should be reasonably efficient. This would apply to all the eliminative channels except the colon as elimination via faeces requires special attention. However, in a world that is not ideal the Lifestyle factors invariably are not managed well at all times resulting in accumulation of toxins at different levels of the body. The recognition of the accumulation of toxins as the biggest contributory cause of illness is absolutely essential.

Medicine today is quite aware of the elimination mechanisms of coughing, sneezing, vomiting, menstruation, and other routes. Unfortunately, not enough attention is given to the evacuation of the colon which leads to so many illnesses.

The re-absorption of water in the digestive tract takes place in the colon. This process of reabsorption of water would invariably result in a film of matter accumulating on the sides of the colon. Normal peristaltic movement does not remove this accumulation which in turn impedes not only subsequent reabsorption but becomes a reservoir for toxic accumulation. The need to keep the colon clean is common to all systems of medicine. They recognize this as a major cause of many symptoms and illnesses, and promote specific treatments which ensure that effective elimination is maintained.

Other Lifestyle Factors

Although the six lifestyle factors described above are the main players in the maintenance of health and healing of disease, they are by no means the only ones.

The following are pertinent to specific individuals and under specific circumstances.

Age and gender

The age and gender of an individual will also have an impact.

Whilst a person's temperament is fixed, (with an ideal qualitative state) the different stages of a person's life from childhood to old age, influences disease conditions that a person may be inclined to. The qualitative changes from infancy to old age are listed on the diagram below.

- **Childhood & teenagers** (Up to 20 years of age): Moist & Hot

- **Youth** (20 to 40 years of age): Hot & Dry

- **Adulthood** (40 to 60 years of age): Cold & Dry

- **Old Age** (From 60 years onward): Cold & moist

The above diagram shows the changes that take place during a person's life cycle from hot and moist to dry and eventually coldness at old age. The qualities associated with each of the stages of the life cycle are an interpretation of the illness conditions that are associated with those stages of life.

Gender refers to the fact that the temperament of females is slightly moister than males with the appropriate inclination towards the respective diseases. For example, more women suffer from depression (which is a disease associated with excess moisture) than men.

Occupation or career

Illnesses which are associated with an individual's career would be specific to that individual. The nature of occupations varies enormously – both physically and mentally. For example, between a young executive sitting behind a desk, in front of a screen all day, with little exercise and no fresh air, and a farm worker out in the sun from dawn to dusk, Also, between an academic, carrying out research, and a manual worker on a car factory production line. Finally, a person may be exposed to toxic or noxious chemicals at work. These can have major effects on a person's health, both over a brief period of time, but more importantly, after chronic exposure over a more extended time span.

Place of residence

This refers to the home environment. This can be overcrowded, which often results in increased tension, aggression and stress. Often ambient noise, lack of ventilation in the home, the presence of insects and house dust mites, can have a deleterious effect on the occupant's health. Also, radioactive gas emanating from the rock underneath is known to be a serious health hazard in certain geological areas.

Exposure to toxic substances

Exposure to pollution in the environment is now considered a major cause of chronic disease in the developed and developing worlds. The source of these pollutants is the enormous number of industrial chemicals, process gases and fumes, nuclear materials, household chemicals, cleaners & detergents. Also important are the numerous additives included processed foods and drinks, the side reaction to the chlorination of water.

Personal habits

Personal habits can also be the direct cause of certain illnesses, or adversely affect existing clinical disorders. Our society is characterised by extensive abusive lifestyle activities. For example, heavy smoking, the use of recreational drugs, spree seasonal or binge drinking, and certain sporting activities. These are not ideal for a person's health.

Pathology in Persian Medicine

Health according to Persian Medicine is the state in which the temperament, ratios of the bodily humors, and bodily structures are in a state of balance, or harmony. In this condition, all the functions in the body perform efficiently and accurately.

An alternative way of describing this is: health is the state based on the complete harmony between the internal and the external environment.

Homeostasis is defined as the tendency of the body's physiological system to maintain an environment of stability. In Persian Medicine homeostasis is described as dynamic optimum functioning. This homeostasis is specific for each individual, and is under the influence of Physis. The maintenance of homeostasis focuses on the person's internal environment, and how it responds to both internal and external stimuli. Physis organizes this balance via the faculties and functions of all the systems and organs of the body, which are under the control of the three main organs – namely, the liver, brain and heart.

The agents of homeostasis are the many physiological systems within the body, such as blood pressure regulation, acid-base balance and body temperature control, which are maintained in equilibrium, in spite of continual variations, both major and minor, in the external environment.

- The homeostasis/harmony we refer to concerns both the inner, internal balance, and its adjustments to the many outside, external influences.

Disease is a disorder of health, with recognizable signs and symptoms which are characteristic of a particular disease. It is diagnosed on the basis of what the physician observes (signs), and what the patient complains of (symptoms). In some cases, diagnostic tests may be necessary to confirm (or reject) the diagnosis.

Disease according to Persian Medicine is that abnormal state of the body in which there is an alteration in the temperamental, humoral, functional and structural level due to any internal or external cause.

In conventional medicine, pathologyis the scientific study of disease processes, with the aim of understanding their nature and causes. It is concerned with the cause, manifestation and diagnosis of a particular disease.

Pathology according to Persian Medicine refers to the state of imbalance (disturbed homeostasis) in the body which tends to affect the body directly. This lack of harmony may be brought about by either internal or external causes. Clinical pathology is the application of the knowledge we have gained from the study of the pathology to the actual treatment of the patient.

Diagnosis is the process of finding out the cause of a patient's medical problem by considering the signs and symptoms, his or her medical history, and any other relevant clinical, social and psychological factors.

The physician's diagnosis may need confirming by observing and testing samples of blood, urine, faeces, sputum and diseased tissue obtained from the living patient or at post-mortem (autopsy), as well as using invasive (endoscopy) or non-invasive imaging (such as X-rays and bone scans).

In Persian Medicine diagnosis includes not only assessing the imbalances at the temperamental, humoral, structural and functional levels but also pays special attention to the patient's unique temperament.

Before we discuss pathology and diagnosis, let us review the importance of maintaining the ideal temperament, because the deviation from this is the underlying cause of all illnesses.

The conventional or allopathic medical understanding of pathology generally involves the following considerations:

Etiology – this is the study of what agent or activity causes a particular disease.

Pathogenesis – this concerns the mechanisms by which a disease originates and develops. Pathogenesis is the basis for prognosis, which is an evaluation of the future course and outcome of a person's ailment.

Morphological changes – this refers to the noticeable changes in tissue or organ structure that develop during the course of the disease.

Clinical significance – Persian Medicine describes the signs and symptoms of the disease. Signs are what the healthcare practitioner observes by use of the five senses. They emerge from the examination. Symptoms are usually the reason for the visit to the healthcare practitioner, or volunteered by the patient on examination or enquiry.

Clinical pathology is the application of the knowledge gained to the treatment of the patient. In Persian Medicine, pathology refers to the state of imbalance, or disturbed homeostasis, in the body which tends to affect the body directly. This lack of harmony may be brought about by both internal and external causes.

Differences between Persian Medicine and conventional methods regarding pathology

There are notable differences in the interpretation of pathology between Persian Medicine and conventional / allopathic medicine.

The main difference is that conventional medicine examines the pathology of a clinical condition by evaluating the disease process in purely physical terms. In particular, it tends to obtain information which is quantifiable or measurable, derived from a wide range of biochemical assays, physiological calculations or imaging techniques. These findings, or parameters, are then interpreted to suggest whether or not there are functional (pathological) or structural (morphological) abnormalities. These findings are based on knowledge of how the disease progressed in other patients in the same age, health and gender bracket.

This approach of obtaining what is measurable and quantifiable has its limitations, as it is purely objective, and operates only at the physical level. It does not take into account the important changes which often take place in the emotional, metaphysical and spiritual dimensions. The reason is simple – these changes cannot be quantified.

Today, conventional medicine is beginning to recognize, to a greater or lesser extent, the effects of these abstract or immeasurable entities. However, it cannot focus on these effectively, as it does not have a philosophical basis for understanding these entities.

Equally important, perhaps, is that what conventional medicine measures, and from which assumptions are being made, is usually more relevant to the final stages of the pathological process. The final stage in the disease process represents only the tip of the iceberg. It is far removed from the origin and early stages of the pathological process.

The Persian Medicine approaches to pathology

The starting point of pathology in Persian Medicine is the ideal qualitative state that is specific to each and every individual. Any change to this ideal beyond the ability of Physis to correct the change will lead to illness.

In Persian Medicine, the understanding of pathology begins at the metaphysical level of the humors and measures outcomes, in terms of the patient's temperament, organ structure and systems function.

Whilst we may not fully comprehend the pathological processes, there is a definite and consistent link between the metaphysical level and the outcomes which can be identified and measured. This tried and tested approach of understanding the causes of illnesses, pathological processes, diagnosis of disease conditions, has proven itself over thousands of years in line with the principles of cause and effect. The fundamentals of pathology in Persian Medicine center around the lack in harmony/homeostasis of the human being as discussed in The Philosophy of Persian Medicine. Pathological processes begin when Physis is unable to maintain homeostasis via the faculties and functions of the systems and organs of the body. This imbalance occurs from the effect of qualities during the interaction between the human being and the environment (represented as the Governing Factors).

In Persian Medicine pathological states are described within the scope of temperament, humors, structure and function under the control of Physis, and in line with the three main organs.

This approach enabled the early practitioners of Persian Medicine to have a comprehensive understanding of outcomes – not only on the pathological process but also within the principles of cause and effect.

- Persian Medicine interprets pathological changes with respect to the relationship between the three main organs and the qualities associated with each organ.

- Pathology in Persian Medicine is not only completely integrative but also acknowledges the causative influences at both (a) the physical level in the tissues and organs, and (b) the metaphysical level, involving changes in humors and qualities.

- Pathological states are described within the concepts of temperament, humors, structure and function, all of which are under the control of Physis.

Persian Medicine and other aspects of pathology

The concept of pathology according to Persian Medicine does not necessarily include purely physiological or biological changes. It focuses rather on the underlying qualitative changes that take place through substantial disturbances in temperament or humors.

The attractiveness of the reasoning behind the conventional approach to pathology can be readily understood. By linking a disorder of an organ or tissue to a particular disease is a simple exercise. In Persian Medicine pathology, however, the symptoms of a particular disease are linked to the distortion in a particular quality.

The physicians who practiced in earlier times were unable to monitor, measure, and understand the millions of biochemical, physiological, and electrical activities within the body. They were, however, able to focus on what can be seen or obtained (signs and symptoms) as well as being able to interpret temperament and humors within the scope of structure and function. Moreover, they had immense metaphysical insights into the workings of the body, in both health and disease.

The three organ theory, shown in the diagram above, may appear to be a very simplistic way of interpreting the complexity of the human body. Yet, it is a very effective and comprehensive system of understanding pathology and diagnosis.

The process from the normal state to the abnormal state

This involves changes in humors, temperament and structure, which ulimately affect metabolic and physiological functions.

Each person's state of normality depends on the ideal qualitative state that is associated with his/her unique temperament at the humoral level. A disturbance in homeostasis will be the inevitable result of a deviation from an individual's ideal qualitative state, in response to a variety of internal or external influences. This deviation will be beyond the ability of Physis to restore this imbalance in a reasonable period of time.

These disturbances can take place along two pathways:

• Temperamental/humoral imbalance: this results in most acute conditions manifesting at a temperamental level. After a prolonged duration, the cause can lead to chronic conditions from a humoral imbalance as well

• Changes in humoral level: this usually results in most chronic conditions.

In both pathways the disease processes develop with imbalances, which lead from temperamental (associated with functional) to humoral or directly from humoral to functional and finally structural imbalances.

Pathway 1: Temperamental/humoral imbalance

In this pathway the changes arise from the onset of a sudden, temporary excess of the qualities heat, coldness, moistness and dryness. These sudden changes or excess of qualities will bring with it the onset of certain symptoms or conditions.

This change in qualities is associated with most acute conditions, and can affect certain functions. The effect of the qualitative changes at a temperamental level, if not reversed, can lead to changes at a humoral level.

InPathway 1, where the cause is a sudden excess qualitative change, Physis can easily restore health once the causative excess quality has been countered. For example, this pathway is common in most cases of self-limiting illnesses, such as colds and flu which affects the respiratory system, and diarrhea, vomiting, and dyspepsia affecting the digestive system.

Pathway 2: Changes at the humoral level

Changes at a humoral level can take place at a quantitative level. This will also affect the qualitative composition of the humors required. Quantitative humoral imbalance arises as a direct result of excess of particular foods which enhance the production of the respective humor. This excess humor will alter the ideal ratio of humors resulting in the two pathological states described below.

Excess humors can cause two pathological states:

1. The excess humor with its particular quality will change the overall quality of the basic humors, so that they are not in

harmony with the qualitative state required by the temperament of the individual. This will lead to a humoral imbalance, with impaired functional consequences.

2. The accumulated excess humor will be prevalent at the vascular level. This will disturb the homeostasis of the internal environment, causing functional disturbances as well as invade tissues and organs, so causing structural damage to tissues and organs.

In either scenario, pathological states can arise from quantitative changes in humors, which can cause either functional imbalance, or cause structural damage or both, so compounding the functional imbalances.

Examples of outcomes of pathways 1 or 2

An outline of illnesses as they progress along Pathway 1 or Pathway 2 will be:

• An example of a *temperamental imbalance* of Cold & Moist qualities can lead to the symptoms which are typical of colds and 'flu, plus their associated functional disturbances such as running nose, cough and bleary eyes. If the effect of these Cold & Moist qualities is prolonged, then this will affect the humoral balance, changing it towards Cold & Moist. For example, this will lead to conditions associated with a phlegmatic (Cold & Moist) humoral imbalance, such as sinus problems, bronchial asthma, bronchitis and even pneumonia, with functional and structural abnormalities (where applicable).

• *Humoral imbalance*, which results from excessive improper diet, will result in qualities of the humors which are not ideal to the person's temperament. Depending on the respective humor that is in excess (with the appropriate quality), that humor will lead to conditions associated with it. For example, an accumulation of the bilious humor can lead to nausea, vomiting, jaundice, hepatitis and gastritis.

Similarly, accumulation of other humors will also result in illnesses associated with that humor.

The invasion of abnormal humors into tissues or organs is invariably as a result of an accumulation of toxins. This is consistent with the wisdom of the early practitioners:

"The ineffective digestion and elimination of the environment is the primary cause of illnesses." *[Hippocrates]*

- All illnesses can be identified into the two pathways, namely, Pathway 1 (mostly acute conditions) or Pathway 2 (mostly chronic ailments).

Relationship of humors to pathology

The changes which occur at a humoral level occur over a period of time. During this period, they can have innumerable outcomes on the functions it will affect, or which organ or tissue it may invade.

All of these possibilities will be dependent on and in line with the group of causes as mentioned in the previous sections, associated with the humors, temperament, and functions. They are dependent to a large extent on the management of the person'sGoverning Factors.

All clinical disorders will:

(a) Either have qualities associated with it, because of a temperamental or a humoral excess, and/or

(a) Arise as a result of damage or structural changes to the affected tissue.

If the clinical condition is associated with an imbalanced humor, the responsible abnormal humor can be easily identified by means of the qualities associated with the condition, as well as the symptoms they present. For example, the accumulation of abnormal bilious humor will be associated with hepatitis (Hot &

Dry), phlegmatic humor with tonsillitis (Cold & Moist) and psoriasis (Cold & Dry).

Foods, humors and disease

As humors are produced from food and drink, the importance and effect of diet on humors and its relationship to associated disease can be appreciated. Obviously diet increasing a specific humor to excess will result in illnesses associated with the respective humor.

Some examples:

- Foods that are Hot & Moist will increase the sanguineous humor.

This may cause or aggravate conditions such as hypertension and dysmenorrhea.

- Foods that are Hot & Dry will increase the bilious humor.

This may cause or aggravate conditions such as hepatitis, pancreatitis, and hyperthyroidism.

- Foods that are Cold & Moist will increase the phlegmatic humor.

This may cause or aggravate conditions such as colds and flu, anemia, and syphilis.

- Foods that are Cold & Dry will increase the melancholic humor.

This may cause or aggravate conditions such as fibrosis, psoriasis, and kidney stones.

The above examples show the influence of diet on humors, which can lead to certain illnesses.

This effect will be as a result of:

(a) the qualities associated with the humors;

(b) The invasion of the humors into the tissues/organs.

- All pathological conditions are the result of a qualitative change, either at the temperamental or the humoral level.

- "You are what you eat"

We have discussed the pathological processes which arise as a result of temperamental or humoral change. We will now discuss the implications of this – namely, the outcome of the pathological process.

The effect of changes in Temperament

If the ideal qualitative state associated with a person's temperament moves from one frame into another (in response to changes in the Governing Factors), the person will be inclined to illnesses of the frame he or she has moved into. This inclination to the illnesses will be dependent on how long the person stays within that frame. This means that a short duration may incline him or her to acute conditions of that frame; a longer duration in the frame will incline him or her to chronic conditions associated with that frame.

Below is an example of an individual who moves from one Qualitative Frame into another, with consequences of the associated illnesses.

Mrs. M has a dominant bilious with a subdominant sanguineous temperament. Being a typical, active, dominant bilious personality she develops endometriosis (a Hot & Dry condition) at the age of 35. By the age of 45, she starts gaining weight, slows down somewhat, and as a result develops hypertension (a Hot & Moist condition). By the age of 50, with increased weight gain, and unable to manage additional worries, her metabolism slows down considerably, and she develops diabetes (a Moist & Hot condition). This gradual movement from one frame into another brings with it the onset of associated illnesses.

The above example highlights the relationship between qualitative changes and the pathological processes, and the clinical implications which follow. It also stresses the importance of adjusting the Governing Factors according to age, so maintaining the ideal temperament. The movement from one Qualitative Frame into another will have a direct bearing on the development of certain illnesses. For example, not respecting the ageing process (which tends to weaken Physis) has pathological implications.

- People will be inclined to illnesses with the Qualitative Frame associated with their temperament.

- Any changes in temperament will result in a movement into another qualitative frame. This will lead to a tendency towards ailments typical of the new frame.

Stages of a particular disease

According to Ibn Sina, there are four distinct stages of an illness or disease:

➢ Commencing Stage – "the beginning"

This stage is the start of the disease, in which the signs and symptoms are not yet prominent, but the disease starts its progress in the body. This arises either from a temperamental or a humoral imbalance. Physis is still relatively in control as there are no apparent signs of functional imbalances.

➢ The Progression Stage – "the increase"

In this stage the disease process accelerates where functional disturbances are apparent and the beginning of structural damage may be evident. Physis is now under pressure to restore the balance with the appropriate systems of the body. This is akin to "orange alert."

➢ The Stage of Crest – "the peak"

The process of increasing of the disease to a peak, Physis is now on "red alert" to overcome the imbalance. During the peak state, the disease can either be:

- Overcome by Physis, so that the body returns to a healthy state.

- Physis succumbs to the disease, and severe chronic disability or death may ensue.

➢ **The Stage of Decline – "the decay"**

The disturbance in the body has been rectified; homeostasis is restored, and health returns.

The above principle applies to all conditions and episodes of illnesses whether they are acute disorders, such as headache and diarrhea, or chronic conditions such as diabetes and asthma.

The role of Physis during pathological processes

Previously we highlighted the fact that the role of the physician is to support Physis.

Throughout the pathological process, from the moment a person moves away from the ideal qualitative state associated with his/her temperament, Physis is doing its best to restore balance. Many pathological states as viewed in conventional medicine are Physis responses which have been brought in to restore the ideal qualitative state of the individual. Symptoms such as sudden fever, sneezing, runny nose, diarrhea and vomiting are regarded as actual ailments - and treated as such - rather considered as a Physis reaction.

Physis not only attempts to restore balance at every step of the disease process, but also acts to minimize the possible damage that might ensue. It achieves this by directing injury towards lesser important organs in order to safeguard the more essential organs. In anaemic conditions, for example, blood circulation will be re-directed for priority use by the key internal organs (brain, heart, liver). This results in the extremities and non-essential organs and tissues receiving less blood than they actually need. They are effectively sacrificed for the sake of the essential organs. Also, if there is an accumulation of toxins in the body, Physis will move the toxins towards the surface of the skin to protect the internal organs. This action is a typical reflex action – very similar to the reflex action when a person protects the head with the hands.

Listed below are some examples of how Physis reacts with either a 'healing response' or with actions which minimize damage.

Healing responses

• An infant refuses food and drink when it is affected by digestive disorders.

• A rise in body temperature occurs, perhaps a fever, when there is a large phlegmatic (Cold & Moist) accumulation. The net effect of this is to facilitate the healing process.

• An increase in heart rate (palpitations) occurs when blood pressure falls to an unacceptably low level, as in shock or when anaemia develops. This action compensates for low blood pressure, so increasing the circulation of blood through the body.

• Perspiration, tears, runny nose, and the build-up of mucus in the upper respiratory and digestive channels occur in the case of hot, spicy foods. This protects the mucous membranes from possible inflammation.

• Increased perspiration develops in febrile conditions. The evaporation of sweat brings the body temperature down, so cooling the body.

• Craving for different tastes and foods (pica) to fulfill a deficiency. For example, the eating of coal or chalk by children and women to compensate for low levels of calcium. Another example is when people with low blood pressure eat saltier foods.

As the increased intake of sodium in salt leads to an increased blood volume, so to a rise in blood pressure.

- The occurrence of vomiting to reject toxins which have been eaten.

- The onset of diarrhea. This serves to expel any possible toxins (contained in foods, or drugs) which may pose a threat to the body.

Responses by Physis to limit damage

- In case of measles and chicken pox, there is a rise in body temperature. This serves to bring the toxic matter to the surface of the skin, thus protecting the internal organs from being damaged.

- Rashes, pimples, itching, eczema, psoriasis and other skin problems develop in order to protect the vital organs from damage. Something like 60% of the offending toxin is excreted through the skin.

- Transient ischemic attack ('mini-stroke') in case of persistently high blood pressure. This is an attempt to prevent the internal organs against damage.

- Recognizing the Physis response, whether it is aimed at healing or for protection, is very important factor in the diagnosis and subsequent treatment of a person's particular ailment.

Summary of pathology from the Persian Medicine perspective

Whilst we may not be able to fully understand every action or response of the body, the philosophical principles of temperament, humors and qualities offer the practitioner distinct advantages.

Persian Medicine enables us to understand the pathological process by interpreting and assessing:

- The causes and progression of a pathological process (temperamental, humoral, functional or structural) and the associated qualities.
- The signs and symptoms presented as a result of the pathological process.
- The qualities associated with the signs and symptoms.
- The qualities associated with the illness condition.
- The Physis response is very important in the diagnosis and treatment of a particular ailment.

Diagnosis in Persian Medicine

A major feature of Persian Medicine is that it highlights the art of diagnosis. Unfortunately, this has been overshadowed in the age we live in, largely because of the extensive dependence on technology. Persian Medicine attaches great importance to meaningful interaction with the patient needed for accurate diagnosis and satisfactory treatment.

The Persian Medicine concept of diagnosis

The art of diagnosis has largely been superseded by a heavy reliance on technology – for biochemical tests (e.g., blood sugar, total cholesterol, liver enzymes) or for physiological parameters (e.g., blood pressure, bone mass index), or for imaging techniques (e.g., gastroscope, X-ray, magnetic resonance imaging).

Conventional medicine focuses sharply on specific parts of the body – diseases of the heart, of the lung, of the kidney, etc. – instead of on the body as a whole. The approach is reductionist, rather than holistic. The picture is further confused by a plethora of detailed chemical parameters. So not surprisingly, not only have healthcare practitioners lost the bigger picture in terms of understanding health; they have also largely lost the art of diagnosis.

Diagnosis involves more than just looking at the results of blood tests, X-rays, chemical and physiological processes in isolation. It needs to realise that all the various relevant components need to be gathered together in relation to the total patient; that is, aspects of the body, the mind and the spirit.

Over and above looking at the patient holistically, the interaction with the patient – listening to the patient, discussing the problem – is equally important. This was evident to the early practitioners.

"It is more important to know what sort of person has a disease than to know what sort of disease a person has" *[Hippocrates]*

The objective of diagnosis

Persian Medicine applies diagnosis in three areas - the symptoms of the condition, the disease itself and the origins (cause) of the disease.

Before one can start with diagnosing any clinical disorder, the practitioner needs first of all to identify the temperament of the individual.

By knowing this aspect of the patient, the practitioner stands to gain valuable insights into the possible causes of the illness, as there is a predisposition to certain illnesses associated with specific temperaments.

Also, by knowing the kind of person the patient is, the practitioner is already empowered with some knowledge which could indicate the possible origin of the disorder. The correlation between the symptoms presented and the temperament of the illness will assist the practitioner in the diagnosis of the condition.

The objectives of the diagnosis are therefore to establish:

- The original temperament of the individual.
- The illness condition.
- The qualities (frames) associated with the illness condition.
- Whether the illness is at a temperamental, humoral, functional or structural level.
- The stage of the progression of the illness (temperamental, humoral, functional, structural).
- The causes of the illness condition (Governing Factors).

The approach to diagnosis in conventional medicine

There is absolutely no doubt that in the field of diagnosis allopathic medicine has made tremendous progress.

Today's technology (electronic stethoscopes, catheterization techniques, biochemical monitoring tests, ultrasound and other imaging techniques, CAT scans, etc.) allows the practitioner to assess biochemical imbalances, and detect and quantify changes at the microscopic level, rapidly and accurately. Over the past fifty years, conventional medicine has appropriately diagnosed (and labeled) illnesses with specific names which encompass symptoms (signs and symptoms), biochemical and physiological imbalances (functions) as well as morphological (structural) changes.

But major elements are missing from this diagnosis–temperament, humors and qualities

If the concept of temperament and humors were applied to the conventional model of diagnosis, then all of the unanswered questions of the causes of illnesses would be taken care of.

Unfortunately, because this dimension is missing, and although the best of hi-tech tools are available, without the inherent wisdom, diagnosis is incomplete.

The approach to diagnosis in Persian Medicine

Simply put, Persian Medicine adopts a holistic approach, integrating available proven clinical modalities, in attempting to identify the cause of the disorder. Once this is achieved, the practitioner is in a position to understand the disorder, and adopt the appropriate healing processes.

Practical guidelines for diagnosis and treatment

"It is more important to know what type of person has a disease than to know what sort of a disease a person has."

Pre-diagnostic evaluation of the patient: Before the standard diagnostic process can get underway, there are a number of important preliminary points which the practitioner needs to be aware of.

- Assess the patient, not the symptoms – treating the patient is more important than addressing the signs and symptoms of the illness.

- Encourage the patient to give an opinion regarding his or her ailment – it will reveal clues as to its origin. It could disclose trigger and aggravating factors, the organs affected, and possibly humoral imbalance. A recurrent headache, for example, may be associated with light, movement, pressure, so help reveal its nature.

- Observe the patient – whilst listening, note the facial coloring, texture and complexion, features of the face and body, speech characteristics, and general body language.

- Request information – ask the patient unobtrusively for more details of his condition or opinion, without interrupting the flow.

Diagnosis of the patient

After the patient has finished commenting on the ailment, then the process of diagnosis can begin. Once the Persian Medicine practitioner has evaluated the signs and symptoms in total, the disease will be largely determined. That is, the nature of the ailment affecting the patient will be placed unequivocally into a "frame of illness".

- Determine the patient's temperament – the Persian Medicine practitioner should differentiate the symptoms from aspects of the patient's temperament. Also ensure that behavior and comments on the patient's condition are not as a result of the condition itself.

- Symptom analysis – the Persian Medicine practitioner should discuss in detail the nature, intensity, frequency and impact of the main symptoms. Note that physical signs and symptoms may be a manifestation of an underlying emotional or spiritual problem.

- Incorrect information – be aware that incorrect information may be proffered by the patient for personal reasons. A common example is the amount and frequency of a patient's alcohol consumption. Another example relates to the patient's smoking habits.

- Assess the patient's emotional state – take note of both positive and negative emotions. A good pointer to the patient's emotional state may be frequent, recurring and intrusive sleep disturbances and dreams.

- Determine the patient's stress level – enquire about stressful life events, both major and minor.

- Note the patient's transition stage – whether he or she is an adolescent, experiencing a mid-life crisis, or is menopausal, for example.

•Look for a connection between symptoms – Somtimes one symptom is a reflection of another. Backache is a good example, as it may be a symptom of not only spinal disorder, but of an abnormal menstrual cycle and even cervical cancer.

•Pay attention to the patient's retention and elimination – this is important, and may be a major factor in subsequent therapy and management.

The ancient healthcare practitioners did not have the technology of today. They therefore had to rely on signs and symptoms of the patient, and diagnose the disorder by using the tools of pulse, urine and stool analysis. However, as they had a comprehensive understanding of temperament and humors they were able to effectively diagnose not only the illness condition, but also the causes of these illnesses.

Diagnosis in Persian Medicine involves not only:

(a) Assessing the ailment with respect to functional and structural imbalances.

(b) Establishing whether the condition is acute (that is, temperament based – associated with qualities) or chronic (humor based).

But also:

(c) The assessment of the temperamental and humoral imbalances themselves.

(d) Determine the cause of the problem by, for example, examining the Governing Factors.

The main approach in the diagnosis, therefore, is to identify the temperamental or humoral imbalance in the patient. This should indicate the possible cause or causes of the condition.

By determining the temperamental and the humoral imbalance, and by observing the functional and structural imbalances (where applicable), the physician would then be able to complete their diagnosis.

Diagnostic procedure

There are four elements to be considered for accurate diagnosis:

(1) Identifying the patient's original temperament

The identification of a person's original temperament will suggest into which frame his ideal qualitative state falls. As discussed earlier, it is the excess qualities of the frames associated with the patient that will invariably affect him the most. Also, the patient will be inclined to the illnesses associated with that frame. However, with changes in qualities (either temperamental or humoral), an individual can move into a frame away from his ideal, even to the opposite extent.

(2) Assess the illness condition.

The illness condition should be assessed by drawing on the Persian Medicine practitioner's experience, intuition and current expertise. Establish whether the condition is acute (that is, temperamental – associated with qualities) or chronic (humoral).

Assess the qualities associated with the illness condition.

As changes in qualities represent the basis of all states of health or disease, identifying the qualities associated with an illness is one of the fundamentals of diagnosis in Persian Medicine.

Using the conditions as appropriate qualities associated with them. These may be the qualities associated with the illness at a temperamental, humoral, functional or structural imbalance. Described in conventional medication at the end of the Section, we have listed all these conditions with the

(4) Determine the cause of the problem, especially with regard to the Governing Factors.

This will require extensive interaction with the patient. The lifestyle and behavior of the patient will need to be clarified in an extensive consultation.

Having identified the condition and the qualities associated with the ailment, one can determine the current frame in which the patient is. Assessing the qualities of the frame the person should be in and comparing this to where he or she is at present will provide clues as to the possible causes, that is, the Governing Factors.

After the diagnosis has been concluded, the signs and symptoms assessed, the patient's history recorded, and the interaction with the Governing Factors determined, the probable cause can be identified.

Symptoms and qualities

Listed below is information regarding symptoms with their associated qualities. The signs and symptoms of a patient were used by the Persian Medicine hakims to establish the qualities associated with the illness as well as to establish the frame in which the illness falls.

Signs and symptoms indicate the qualities associated with an imbalance, whether it is at a temperamental or humoral level. These signs and symptoms are what the patients present externally, so can be interpreted by assessing the functional and structural changes that take place which deviate from the normal health state.

It is important to note that the Persian Medicine concept of symptoms and disease conditions differ in perspective from that of conventional medicine. For example, in allopathic medicine vomiting or diarrhea are defined as discrete illness conditions. However, in Persian Medicine these phenomena are considered as symptoms (or signs) which indicate either

(a) A Physis response to the need for eliminating undigested food or

(b) An accumulation of phlegmatic humor in the gastrointestinal tract.

In addition, there are times when a patient may present with symptoms which may not be associated with the same Qualitative Frame. For example, a person who suffers from hypertension (which is located within the Hot & Moist frame) may develop colds & flu symptoms which are actually associated with the Cold & Moist frame. Indeed, these anomalies of distant frames or even opposite frames may be present in a patient at the same time.

What will be invariably found is that most of the chronic illnesses associated with the individual will be those into which his/her temperament falls.

Acute conditions, on the other hand, can be from any of the other Qualitative Frames. In general, however, there will be consistency with the symptoms or illness conditions associated with the Qualitative Frames.

Effect of excess qualities

The signs and symptoms of particular ailments follow on from the effects of the four qualities of heat, moistness, dryness and coldness. The effects of these are mentioned below, followed by symptoms with the corresponding qualities in the six Qualitative Frames as well as the qualities associated with illness conditions.

(1) Quality of Heat

Excessive heat causes:

- A decrease in moistness resulting in an increase of dryness.

- An imbalance in the sanguineous humor.

- Stimulation of the bilious humor (heat and dryness).
- A decrease in the phlegmatic humor.

(2) Quality of Coldness

Excessive coldness causes:

- An increase in the phlegmatic humor.
- A decrease in heat resulting in an imbalance between bilious and sanguineous humors.
- An increase in the melancholic humor.

(3) Quality of Moistness

Excessive moistness causes:

- A decrease in heat results in an imbalance in the bilious and sanguineous humors.
- A decrease in dryness.
- An increase in the phlegmatic humor.

(4) Quality of Dryness

Excessive dryness causes:

- An imbalance in the sanguineous humor.
- A decrease in moistness resulting in a decrease in the phlegmatic humor.
- All signs, symptoms as well as illness conditions have qualities associated with them.
- All illness conditions can be placed into one of the six Qualitative Frames.

- Symptoms may not always fall in the same frame with respect to a particular patient.

Diagnosis

Introduction

Diagnosis is the heart of the medical art; it is what separates medicine as a definite, rational science from medical magic and superstition. Diagnosis is also the central, golden link in the chain of medical knowledge that brings together all its theoretical aspects to provide the practical key to treatment. Diagnosis, to be accurate and sound, must be built upon a broad yet definite base of knowledge regarding all aspects of human anatomy, physiology and pathology.

Knowledge of anatomy will enable the physician to spot and correct any deviations or abnormalities in the structure of body parts, organs or tissues and use them as clues to pathology.

Knowledge of physiology or the normal, righteous functioning of the body will help the physician to recognize and pinpoint pathological deviations from it, and to identify exactly what needs to be restored. In Persian Medicine, all physiological concepts are based on the Seven Natural Factors, which are discussed in the Basic Principles section.

Knowledge of pathology, or how the normal, healthy structure and function of the body becomes altered and deranged by disease, enables the physician to identify these morbid changes and deviations when he sees them in his patient. In Persian Medicine, pathology involves deviations in one or more of the Seven Natural Factors (see above), as well as negligence in one or more of the Six Essential Factors, which are described and discussed in the Health Preservation section; violation of hygiene is the most common cause of pathology.

In addition, there is one other essential ingredient to accurate, effective diagnosis that enables the physician to make proper use of all the technical medical knowledge described above. And that's knowledge of philosophy, which clarifies the physician's powers of reasoning and deduction, and enables him to distinguish the underlying truth behind only surface appearances. This is why Avicenna considered philosophy to be a central, essential part of the physician's training.

In conclusion, proper diagnosis is the key to all effective medical treatment. The more precise and accurate your diagnosis, the more specific and effective will be the treatment. You can't fix something properly unless you know exactly what is wrong, or out of order.

Diagnosis: Tradition versus Modern

The practice of diagnosis in modern medicine has been totally altered by the advance of high technology. The modern physician relies heavily on technology and sophisticated machinery throughout the diagnostic process: EEGs, EKGs, diagnostic scanners and imaging equipment, radiography and lab tests.

The physician had none of that to fall back on. He had nothing but his five senses and a few simple diagnostic tools, like a stethoscope or a reflex hammer.

This lack of outer equipment made it essential for the physician to train his inner, human instrument - his mind, and his five senses - fine them to a high degree of perfection.

In the modern diagnostic process, with its heavy reliance on technology and machinery, there is a danger that these diagnostic skills and sensitivities can become atrophied from disuse. Also, the modern medical environment tends to favor an exclusive reliance on quantitative data that can be numbered and measured as the only information that's really reliable and trustworthy; the qualitative data and observations used in more forms of medical diagnosis tend to be discounted.

For example, the traditional physician would observe a patient's yellowish or sallow complexion and conclude, along with other signs and symptoms, that he/she was suffering from jaundice, or a bilious disorder. The modern physician wouldn't be content with that qualitative observation alone, and would order lab tests to quantify raised levels of bilirubin or liver enzymes before arriving at that conclusion.

In all traditional medical systems, the diagnostic model used in that system is based on the basic physiological and pathological concepts of that system. The therapeutic system and modalities of treatment offered by that same traditional medical system are also keyed in to these same basic pathophysiological concepts.

For example, black bile, or the Melancholic humor, exists as a pathophysiological concept or clinical entity in Persian Medicine, and diagnostic conclusions are based on it. And Persian Medicine also has reliable medicines and tools in its therapeutic for correcting disorders and imbalances of black bile.

Modern medicine may protest that black bile doesn't really, objectively exist, and perhaps it actually doesn't. But for all practical purposes, clinically useful diagnoses can be arrived at and effective treatment strategies can be designed and carried out based on the pathophysiological concept of black bile.

Besides constant practice in the traditional diagnostic techniques, the physician often works to sharpen and hone the sensitivity of his senses through meditation and special exercises. In addition, meditation also develops the physician's powers of insight and intuition.

Whereas modern medicine tends to be quite literal and concrete in its approach to diagnosis, healing systems like Persian Medicine tend to take a more poetic, figurative approach. Through the tongue, pulse or other diagnostic signs, the patient's body is trying to communicate to the physician what is wrong with it; the physician's job is to learn the language of the patient's signs and symptoms, listen to them, and get the message.

Signs, Symptoms and Syndromes

Avicenna countered that a complete diagnostic assessment required a consideration of both the patient's signs and symptoms.

A symptom is what the patient tells the physician about how he or she feels - feelings of pain, discomfort, hunger, thirst, nausea, or anything strange or abnormal. Symptoms are the subjective feelings and sensations of the patient about his/her condition.

A sign is an objective phenomenon observed or diagnosed by the physician in the patient. A rapid pulse, contracted "pinpoint" pupils, or red, bloodshot eyes would be examples of signs. Certain signs can be diagnostic of certain diseases. Avicenna was the first to systematize, prioritize, and correlate the various signs and symptoms found in different diseases, and give explanations as to what might be causing them. And so, Avicenna virtually founded the art of differential diagnosis.

Avicenna approached the art of diagnosis holistically, taking the entire organism - body, mind and spirit - to be one indivisible whole, or physis. Since the whole organism is responding in a unified manner to the challenge of disease, Avicenna was the first to recognize that signs or symptoms appearing in one part of the body could be indicative of a disease process happening in another distant part of the body.

A syndrome is, literally, a certain constellation of associated signs and symptoms that" run around together". Some of these sign - symptom constellations are indicative or diagnostic of certain diseases, whereas other syndromes have yet to be fully explained or linked to a definite pathology or disease. Nevertheless, Persian Medicine recognizes that many syndromes can be successfully treated and resolved, even though their pathological and causative mechanisms aren't fully known.

Methods of Diagnosis

The traditional physician had to be very perceptive and resourceful in using all his five senses, and whatever was at his disposal in diagnosing disease, and assessing the patient's condition. Above all, the first and most important method of diagnosis was taking a good medical history in the initial patient intake process, and then following up with one's careful observations of the patient and the disease as it develops and progresses.

Visual diagnosis includes careful observation and inspection of the patient's general behavior, spirit and posture and physique; skin color, or complexion; facial signs, eyes and physiognomy; nails, tongue, hair, etc...

Palpation or tactile diagnosis obviously includes pulse diagnosis, as well as palpating the chest and abdominal cavities. It involves feeling heat or coldness, softness or hardness, dryness or moisture, and fullness or emptiness.

Auscultation, or auditory diagnosis includes listening to the patient's voice or breathing sounds; using a stethoscope to listen to the patient's heartbeat, gastrointestinal or lung sounds; and percussion of the chest and abdomen to listen for either hollow, resonant or dull sounds.

Olfaction can also be used to smell the patient's breath or body odor, as well as odors of any of the bodily secretions or excreta.

The bodily excreta are important diagnostic indicators in themselves that also deserve careful inspection and study. Excretion, or elimination, is the final stage of pepsis, or digestion and metabolism. You can tell a great deal about the body's metabolic processes by what they excrete as superfluous or unusable waste. The main excreta that are inspected for diagnostic purposes are the urine and the stool. Persian Medicine is especially known for its urine diagnosis, although the stool is also important.

There are some masters physicians that have developed such consummate skill in a particular diagnostic technique, like the pulse, that no further information is needed for an accurate diagnosis than hearing the patient's chief complaint and taking his/her pulse. But for the majority of physicians, especially beginning practitioners of the medical art, forming a broad, composite picture from many different diagnostic methods is the surest way to arrive at an accurate diagnosis.

Taking a medical history

Taking a medical history is the heart of the diagnostic process in Persian Medicine. The medical history is the grand centerpiece, the big picture that provides a panoramic overview of the patient's entire illness or health condition - how it originated, how it grew and developed, and how it is at present.

It is primarily the medical history that tells the physician which specific signs to check for, and what other forms of diagnosis are needed to obtain the information he seeks. And so, all other methods of diagnosis can be seen as auxiliaries to the medical history, which is the principal, or core diagnostic method.

The medical history also has certain distinctive features and attributes that are essential and not found in other diagnostic methods. First, the medical history covers the past tense, or the genesis and development of the patient's various illnesses and complaints. Secondly, the medical history and patient interview is the main vehicle for eliciting information about the patient's subjective symptoms; how the patient reacts to, experiences, or feels about his/her illness may be just as important as, or more important than, the illness itself, and provide valuable keys to treatment.

Doctor - Patient Relationship

In Persian Medicine, the medical history and dialogue between the patient and his/her physician is the heart of the doctor - patient relationship. It is here that the physician establishes a rapport with his patient, and communicates to him/her his sincere caring and commitment to their recovery and improvement of health and wellbeing. This caring in itself can have great therapeutic value.

Sadly, this personal rapport between doctor and patient is what is most lacking in modern medicine. On the average, it is said that the modern doctor spends only about ten minutes or so talking to his patient. This cold impersonality of modern medicine can be anti-therapeutic, and exacerbate the problem.

The success of the medical history and patient interview depends on the good communication skills of the physician. To avoid getting a biased or one-sided account from the patient, the physician must learn to ask unbiased, open-ended questions; he must also, both verbally and nonverbally, learn how to evoke an atmosphere of openness, trust, and cooperation from his patient. The physician must learn how to bring his vast knowledge of physiology and pathology into play by asking the right questions at the right times, to get the information he most needs to know to differentially diagnose and treat the patient's condition. The physician must elicit the desired information clearly and unambiguously from his patient.

Patients want a doctor who is sympathetic and caring, who listens to them and validates their needs and concerns; they also want a doctor who is open, frank and honest in his dealings with them. The physician must also radiate energy of cheerfulness and enthusiasm, and make the patients feel good about them, which is half the battle in healing. The physician must be skilled in human relations, being the right thing at the right time to the right people, as the situation demands.

The physician in Persian Medicine is, above all, a teacher and way shower, a Natural Philosopher; he must teach health and healing not just by his verbal instructions to the patient, but also by his own personal example. The physician is a personal guide, coach, mentor, counselor and resource person to his patient, making his healing wisdom freely accessible to all who seek his help. The patient's healing and recovery are more complete and lasting if the physician not only prescribes treatments and medicines, but also instructs the patient in the art of healthy living.

The Basic Structure of the Medical History

In all medical systems, the basic format and structure of the medical history and patient interview is patterned after the basic theoretical concepts of that system. In this, Persian Medicine is no exception.

After taking the patient's name, age, sex and other basic data, the thing that starts the medical interview or patient intake process is the patient's chief complaint. The chief complaint is whatever brought the patient in to seek the physician's help.

After the chief complaint come the patient's various subsidiaries or auxiliary complaints. These may be closely related to the chief complaint, or they may not be. Somtimes, and actually quite often, the chief complaint, or what brings the patient in to see the doctor, may not actually be the patient's most serious complaint, or disorder. This is due either to ignorance and confusion, or to a distorted ranking of values and priorities on the part of the patient. After this come inquiries into the patient's dietary, hygiene or lifestyle habits as possible causes or contributors to the patient's health problems and concerns. In Persian Medicine, these inquiries are structured according to the Six Essential Factors: ambient air, food and drink, exercise and rest, sleep and wakefulness, retention and evacuation of wastes, and perturbations of the mind and emotions.

Then, a general review of systems is in order. This is done first according to signs and symptoms of aggravations of the Four Humors, then physiologically and pathologically, according to the Four Faculties and their various organ systems.

After this comprehensive inquiry and review are finished, then the patient is asked to inquire about any remaining health problems or concerns; these may give valuable clues and leads concerning things that were missed in previous portions of the medical history. Somtimes, in light of this final dialogue, the physician may also be moved to ask specific questions regarding that which avoid him earlier.

The Chief Complaint

The chief complaint is what brings the patient in to see the doctor. It's the initial point of departure for the medical history, and everything unfolds from the patient's description of the chief complaint.

The physician usually starts the dialogue with a simple, "What can I do for you?", or "What's been bothering you?" The physician should make this initial inquiry as broad, neutral and open-ended as possible, allowing the patient unlimited latitude in describing the chief complaint as he/she sees it.

After the chief complaint has been described, the physician should inquire about its severity, and whether it is constant or intermittent. If intermittent, the physician should try to ascertain the frequency of attacks, or onsets. In particular, the severity of any pain, if present, should be precisely ascertained and described.

After the nature and scope of the chief complaint have been thoroughly ascertained, the physician should inquire about the time and manner of its origin or onset, and how it developed into its present state. The physician should try to ascertain as much as possible about the various factors and circumstances that led to the onset and development of the chief complaint.

Then, what's very important is to ask questions like, "What makes it worse / brings it on?" and, "What makes it better / provides relief?" These two questions adjusted or modified depending on whether the chief complaint is constant or intermittent. The patient's responses to these questions may provide valuable clues as to the nature and temperament of the patient's illness or condition.

Auxiliary Complaints

With a simple, "What else is bothering you?" or, "Is there anything else I should know about?" the physician elicits information from the patient regarding any subsidiary or auxiliary complaints that he/she may be experiencing.

The physician should then do a workup of each subsidiary or auxiliary complaint in much the same manner as for the chief complaint. The dimensions to be ascertained are: its degree, or severity; its time and circumstances of onset; its manner of growth and development; and its modalities, or various aggravating or palliating factors.

Somtimes, these other complaints may be directly related to the chief complaint, in which case it is called a subsidiary complaint. If it developed as a direct consequence or outgrowth of the chief complaint, the subsidiary complaint is called a complication.

Somtimes, these other complaints may bear very little connection, if any, to the chief complaint, appearing to be totally independent and unrelated. In these cases, it would be called an auxiliary complaint. However, much independence and autonomy an auxiliary complaint may appear to have from the chief complaint, there's always some connection.

Since the underlying biological and metabolic terrain prevailing in the patient's body is one and the same, there are always some common themes shared by these various complaints that indicate the basic nature and temperament of this terrain.

The physician should always ascertain the relative chronological order in which the patient's various illnesses and complaints had their onset, and then developed. This will tell the physician which of the patient's disorders are primary, and the most chronic and deep-seated, and which are secondary, being consequences, complications of the original complaint.

All of the patient's various illnesses, complaints and disorders fit together into one big composite picture of the patient's overall condition. In various holistic healing systems, the patient's original or most chronic, deep-seated complaints are likened to the roots or trunk of a tree, whereas the secondary complications are likened to a tree's branches, or to the fruit that the tree bears.

Whatever the analogy used, the fact is that the whole picture of the patient's condition and its various complaints, or pathological manifestations, in their relative severity and chronological sequence of development, is as unique and distinctive to that patient as his/her fingerprint. In disease and pathology, as well as in constitution and physiology, each patient is a unique individual.

Usually, the patient's chief complaint is the most serious disorder he/she faces, but, surprisingly often, it's not, and one of the other complaints reveals itself to be the root problem or condition, the most serious and deep-seated. This may indicate either ignorance or lack of awareness on the patient's part, or it may actually be due to a confused, disordered or inappropriate system of values and priorities, as in a preoccupation with weight loss and surface appearance when serious underlying health problems exist. Hopefully, in these cases, the physician can re-educate and re-orient the patient towards a healthier arrangement of values and priorities.

Tongue and Pulse

It is here, after a thorough workup and evaluation of the patient's chief and subsidiary / auxiliary complaints has been done, that the time is right for taking the patient's pulse and looking at his/her tongue. The tongue and pulse are important barometers as to the basic nature and temperament of the patient's condition, and the pathogenic factors that are causing the patient's various symptoms and complaints. Often, the tongue and pulse will suggest or indicate important lines of questioning that will turn up new diagnostic information and complaints.

Constitutional Assessment and Family History

By this point in the patient interview, the physician practitioner of Persian Medicine should definitely have formed some impression of the patient's constitutional nature and temperament. This will be evident not just from the patient's account of his/her various symptoms and complaints in response to the physician's inquiries, but also from visual impressions of the patient's physiognomy, physique, complexion, behavior, vitality level and mannerisms. These initial impressions can later be altered or modified by data collected in the subsequent parts of the medical history.

At this point, it's a good time to ask the patient about diseases that run in his/her family. Since one's native constitution is generally inherited from one's parents, such family diseases are often good indicators of the patient's constitutional type and its predispositions.

It's also a good idea for the physician to prepare a form, checklist or questionnaire that the patient fills out beforehand to define more precisely his/her constitutional nature and temperament. This questionnaire can be constructed based on the Four Temperaments.

Constitutional nature and temperament can also be determined through the pulse, for more information on pulse and temperament. If the practitioner's proficiency in pulse diagnosis is not yet advanced enough to precisely pinpoint the patient's constitutional nature and temperament, it can provide valuable clues and leads in this direction.

The Six Essential Factors

A review of the patient's daily habits of diet, hygiene and lifestyle is essential to any good medical history. In Persian Medicine, this portion of the medical history is structured after the Six Essential Factors.

This portion of the medical history is important for two main reasons: First, errors in diet, hygiene and lifestyle are major causative factors in the majority of diseases, especially the chronic and degenerative diseases so prevalent today. Secondly, information on the patient's daily habits of diet, hygiene and lifestyle provides important clues as to the nature of the patient's physiology and metabolism, and his/her constitutional nature and temperament. With this portion of the medical history, we often uncover causative factors behind the patient's illnesses and complaints that were previously obscure.

So, here are the Six Essential Factors, and the main inquiries the physician needs to make in relation to each:

Ambient Air: Respiratory problems, difficulty breathing, shortness of breath. Expectoration, phlegm discharges, Seasonal allergies. Living environment- its ventilation and exposure to the elements: sunlight, wind, dryness, rain, dampness, etc., Air purity and pollution levels, the country, climate and terrain.

Food and Drink: A typical meal menu for breakfast, lunch and dinner, Meal frequency and regularity; skipped meals, Meal scheduling, favorite foods and drinks, Problematic foods and drinks, Food allergies and sensitivities, Meat consumption and its effects, Dairy consumption and its effects, Consumption of fresh fruits and vegetables, Fluid and water consumption, hydration levels, Dietary supplements and herbs taken. Digestive problems, symptoms and/or discomforts after eating, such as sluggishness, somnolence, gas, distension, bloating, etc...

Exercise and Rest: General degree of sedentariness versus activity, Frequency and duration of vigorous exercise and physical activity per week. Favorite sports and recreational activities, Aerobic and cardiovascular capacity, Endurance levels, Athletic performance, Fatigue, stress, trauma or injury after exercise, Athletic injuries, muscular aches and pains. Ability to rest, recover and rebound adequately after exercise.

Sleep and Wakefulness: Sleep habits - duration and scheduling of sleep, time to bed and time to raise (average), Soundness and regenerative capacity of sleep, Tendency towards insomnia or excessive sleep and somnolence, Nature and character of dreams; incidence or frequency of troubled or disturbing dreams, Daytime napping. Energy levels in general, and throughout the day.

Retention and Evacuation of Wastes: This is a particularly important area, as Avicenna considered autointoxication from retained toxins, wastes and morbid humors to be the primary causative factor in most diseases. Constipation has been called the Mother of All Diseases. However, excessive evacuation and an inability to adequately hold on to wastes are also pathological.

There are four major bodily wastes in Persian Medicine, and pertinent inquiries are made about each:

Sweat: Easy or excessive sweating, Spontaneous or furtive sweating, even without undue heat or physical activity. Complete absence of sweating, or inability to sweat, Sweating from nervousness or stress. Burning or itching sweat, Heat rashes, and Hot flashes. Night sweats.

Exhalation: Excessive yawning, Stuffy chest, constricted breathing, Excessive sighing, Bad breath.

Urine: Urine frequency and volume, Urine color, Frequent, urgent or painful urination, Gravel or sediment, Difficulty passing urine. See Urine Diagnosis page for details.

Stool: Frequency of defecation, and size of stool. Stool hardness, softness, texture, consistency, Color of stool, Presence of diarrhea or soft stools, Alternating constipation and diarrhea, irritable bowel.

Perturbations of the Mind and Emotions: General mental and emotional outlook, Relationships, sex, love life, marital relations, Relations with children, offspring, Relations with bosses, coworkers. Job related stress. Stress in general. Note patient's mannerisms, general behavior, and body language.

A Review of Humors, Faculties and Systems

As part of the initial intake process, the patient can check off items on a check list. This will save the physician time when taking the medical history, as he only needs to focus on and inquire further about items the patient checked as being applicable to him/her. For each of the complaints or conditions checked, the physician needs to inquire at least about its general frequency and severity; if he feels that the symptom, condition or complaint is important, the physician may go into more detail about it with the patient.

The first section of this checklist should consist of four groups or columns of symptoms, with each group pertaining to common symptoms associated with the aggravation or plethora of a certain humor. The second part of this form should have common symptoms and complaints listed according to faculty and organ system.

Conclusions and Diagnosis

Finally, there should be space on the patient intake and history form for the physician to draw up his conclusions about the patient's overall condition, and formulate a working diagnosis. This is the end towards which the physician is striving, through all the signs, symptoms and other diagnostic information that he takes in. If the medical history has been orderly and thorough, and the right supplemental methods of diagnosis have been used where necessary and indicated, the right diagnostic conclusions should naturally fall into place.

Identifying temperament

Clinically, a person's temperament can be diagnosed using the following ten criteria:

1. Touching

The temperament of a person is diagnosed by comparing the feel of his body with the normal person under equable climatic and atmospheric conditions. If feel is the same in both cases the temperament is balanced, however, it may be relatively hot or cold. Somtimes the softness, roughness and dryness of finger nails help to reveal the temperament provided it has not resulted from some extraneous cause.

the conclusion drawn from a soft or hard feel defined upon the proper balance of heat and cold (in the body) because excess of heat after dispersing the moisture make the body soft and moist even when it was originally hard. Cold makes the normal or even soft body hard as in the ice. This may cause some confusion persons of cold temperament; generally, feel soft even though they are this and well. This is an account of the excess of immature humors.

2. Muscularity and Adiposity

A good muscular development indicates greater heat and moisture in the body. In such cases the body feel find solid to touch. Poor muscular development and deficiency of fat indicate dryness. Excess of fat and oiliness (of skin) point to the moisture temperament. In such case the body feels soft and flabby.

The deficiency or excess of fat in the body, however, depends upon the excess or deficiently of the muscularity and the temperament is likely to be hot and moist. When both solid and liquid fats are abundant there is excess of cold and moisture in the body and thus a cold and most temperament is existing.

3. Hair

The signs pertaining to hair are; rapidity or slowness of growth, excess or scantiness, thinness or thickness, straightness or curliness and colors.

Slow growth or lack of growth is a sign of excessive moisture if there are no interfering factors such as anemia; malnutrition etc. rapid growth of hair is a sign of dryness. Heat and dry when present the hair becomes thick and profuse and grows more rapidly. This is due to rapid growth results from excess of heat while thickness from excess of smoke (metabolic products), hence adult's hair is coarse but of children is fine because they have less smokiness and more moisture. Scanty hair is a sign of the cold and moist temperament.

Dark color pertains to a hot and brown to cold temperament. Tawny hair denotes a balanced temperament. grey hair pertains to a cold and moist temperament as in old people some time grey hair is a sign of extreme dryness as in the cause of plants which lose their dark green color and turn which an account of dryness. This happens also in the dry group of diseases. According to Aristotle, hair turns grey because of phlegm. It must be remembered that the color of hair in influenced by habitat and climate. In youth, color of hair is similar to that of the people in southern countries, while the color in child hood in likes that of the people in northern countries. During middle age color of hair resembles that of the people living in the central region.

Excess of hair is a sign of excessive black bile in elderly persons it is, however, a sign of black bile being already excessive.

4. Complexion

Pallor denotes loss for deficiency of blood and therefore, a cold temperament. If with deficient blood there is heat or excess of bile, the complexion is yellow and not pale. Rosy complexion indicates excess of heats well as more blood while the yellow and blond colors refer to excess of simple heat. Yellow complexions; however, indicates excess of bile while a blonde complexion pertain to excess of blood or bilious. Occasionally, as convalescents, yellow color may be the result of anemia rather than excessive bile. A bluish tongue denotes to excess of cold. It is an indication that there is less blood formation and whatever little blood in from is being congealed and thus becomes dark. Wheal complexion is a sign of heat while purple color denotes cold and dryness from the excess of black bile. Chalky color is a sign of cold and phlegm. Ivory complexion pertains to a small quantity of bile being mixed in the cold phlegm. The type of complexion is found in disorders of the liver while dark yellow color is generally seen in disorders of the spleen. Color of the tongue is an excellent guide to the temperamental conditions of blood vessel both the pulsating arteries as well and the quiescent veins color of eyes is a reliable indication of the temperament condition of brain. Somtimes, in the same disease, color of organ may differ from that of the other for example, in the case of excessive combustion of bile, the tongue is white but the face is dark.

5. Physique

Persons of hot temperament have blood chests, with large and well developed but not small and narrow hands and feet. The blood vessels are prominent and of wide caliber and pulse generally strong and of large volume. These people have good muscular development especially around the joints. This is because growth and development are carried out by heat. Persons of cold temperament have the opposite characteristics because cold hinders the growth and functional maturity of organs. The characteristics of dry temperaments are dryness and roughness of the skins, prominence of joints, thinness and prominence of nasal and tracheal cartilages and an erect nose.

6. Sleep and Wakefulness

Natural sleep and wakefulness are signs of normal balance particularity in brain. Excessive sleep denotes undue cold and moisture while excess of wakefulness refers to excess of heat and dryness especially in the brain.

7. Functional state of organs

As long as the functions are performed in a natural well integrated and "whole" manner, the temperament is well balanced. Over active and exaggerated functions, such as rapid growth and movements, indicate excess of heat e.g. rapid development of organs, growth of hair and quick eruptions of teeth. Weakness and sluggish mass of functions is a sign of cold temperament. A hot temperament can also produce weak and sluggish movements. In the results of associated weakness, several physiological functions are lost or impaired by heat e.g. loss or reduction of sleep. On the other hand, some physiological activities are increased by cold e.g. steep. Sleep is however, not absolutely and independently physiological but is necessary. It is not for its own sake but because it gives the vital force rest from exhausting activities. Sleep enables the vital force to devote its undivided attention to digestion. This is not possible in wakefulness which is inverse activities. It is thus clear that sleep is indispensable and thus natural. A phenomenon which is indispensable is natural by virtue of necessity.

Functions are reliable indication of temperaments. When they are normal and healthy, the temperament is balanced. Entrances of hot, cold, dry, and most temperament for the functional state of organs is however, a rough guide. Functions which point to heat are blood and powerful voice, continuous and rapid speech, short temper, brisk movements and frequent blinking. They are signs not only of general heat in the body but also of heat in the corresponding organs.

8. Excretions

The conditions of excretions stool, urine and sweat also indicate the temperament state of the body. Thus strong odors, high color, full maturity and proper consistency of excretions are signs of heat. The opposite features denote coldness of temperament.

9. Passivity of the four qualities

As a role excessive passivity to one of the main domain quality, hot or cold, means that the person or the organ has the same temperament.

10. Psychological Activity

The sign of heat pertaining to the actions and reaction of psyche are: intensity of anger, depth of sadness and sorrow, cuteness of perception and memory, excessive initiative, lack of scruples, over trust, optimism, callousness, vigilance, manliness, active habits, insensitivity and slowness reactions.

A cold temperament is characterized by offsite qualities. Persistence of joy or anger and good memory indicate dryness wile forgetfulness is a sign of excessive moisture.

dreams also paint to the nature of temperament e.g. dreams of sitting near the five, or bathing in the sum paint to heat while feeling of chillness and of being submerged in cold water suggest a cold temperament. Dominances of various humors have their own characteristic dreams.

All or at least, majority of the signs mentioned above are diagnostic of the innate and congenital temperaments.

Each person is unique. Just as we have a unique fingerprint, so we have a unique temperament

Summary of the sign of balanced temperament

The sign of balanced temperament selected from amongst the signs described above are summarized as follows:

1. Feel of the body is balanced in respect of heat, cold dryness, moisture, softness and hardness

2. Complexion ranges between pallor and redness.

3. Body build is neither too heavy nor too lean.

4. Blood vessels are neither superficial nor prominent none deeply submerged and hidden.

5. Hair is neither profuse non scanty and neither too think and dark of maturity.

6. Sleep and wakefulness are moderate.

7. Movements are free and easy.

8. Intellectual powers and memory are good.

9. Habits and behavior are balanced between courage and timidity, anger and calmness, callousness and leniency, ready violence and quality dignity, pride and humility.

10. Functions of all organs in the body are "whole" and correct.

11. Growth is rapid and deterioration of faculties slows.

12. Dream is interesting and pleasing and portrays cheerful and pleasant company with sweet voices and fragrant surroundings

13. Good humor, popularity and geniality are fairly characteristic.

14. Meals are enjoyed and consumed is moderation and digested and assimilated normally.

15. Excretory functions are regular and normal.

Pulse diagnosis

Of all the traditional diagnostic methods, none is more legendary than pulse diagnosis. With nothing more than hearing the patient's chief complaint and taking his/her pulse, the master of pulse diagnosis can arrive at a complete and accurate diagnosis of the patient's condition.

Avicenna discusses pulse diagnosis extensively in volume I of the Canon of Medicine, which has become the basic clinical manual for practitioners of Persian Medicine.

The great virtue and advantage of pulse diagnosis is that it enables the physician to read this River of Life in real time, and perceive directly the action of the vital principles, the condition of the humors, internal organs and their physiological functions as they happen. Taking a medical history covers the origins, history and development of the patient's condition, but pulse diagnosis presents it in the present moment, in dynamic, kinetic motion.

What is the Pulse?

The arteries are rooted in the heart, the principal organ of the Vital Faculty. With each beat or pulsation, the heart infuses the blood with the vital principles: The Innate Heat and Vital Force.

Because the arteries are seamlessly connected to and extensions of, the heart, with each contraction or beat of the heart, the arteries pulsate. Because the arteries carry fresh blood infused with the vital principles to every cell, organ and tissue of the body, you could say that the arteries pulsate as an expression of the Vital Force they contain.

Blood is the gross, humoral vehicle for the subtle vital energies - the Innate Heat and Vital Force. The flow of the Vital Force guides the circulation of the blood, and in the healthy body, they run seamlessly together in perfect union and harmony. In certain pathological conditions, however, the blood and the Vital Force can fall out of sync, or out of balance with one another, which is apparent in the pulse.

There are two phases of the heartbeat, or cardiac cycle: contraction, or systole; and relaxation, which is diastole. With each systole, or heart contraction, blood is pumped out of the heart into the arteries, which swell, or rise. With each diastole, or heart relaxation, blood enters the heart, easing pressure on the arteries, which deflate, or fall.

And so, the pulse rises with each systole, and falls with each diastole of the heart. The relative quality, feel and discreteness of the arterial rises and falls are another dimension of pulse reading. Avicenna also tells us that there are pauses or transitional phases between the rise of systole and the fall of diastole, the quality and discreteness of which can also be read and interpreted.

The Technique of Pulse Taking

There are many different arteries at which the pulse can be felt. But in Persian Medicine and most other medical systems, the radial artery at the wrist, just medial to the radius bone and proximal to the thumb, on the prone side of the wrist, is used.

Taking the pulse at the radial artery has several distinct advantages:

A relatively long stretch of artery is exposed, lying close to the surface, for easy palpation in many positions.

The artery can be easily presented to the physician, without difficulty, discomfort, or distress.

The radial artery branches out fairly closely and directly from the heart, receiving a strong flow and pulsation of blood. It is also in the middle part of the body, not too high and not too low, and therefore is representative of the whole organism and all its major organs.

The physician's middle finger is placed on the radial artery, directly across from the prominence of the radius bone, with the other three adjacent fingers falling naturally right next to it. In the Persian Medicine method, the index finger lies closest to the heart.

Ideally, the pulse should be taken on an empty stomach, and not immediately after eating. It also should not be taken when angry, upset or tired; after a bath; or after sex.

Basic Qualities or Parameters of the Pulse

There are certain basic qualities or parameters of the pulse that are obvious and immediately apparent to anyone who has ever felt the pulse. The clinical significance of these various qualities is that they are similar qualities or states prevailing within the organism. These basic qualities or parameters are:

- Speed, also known as frequency.
- Force, also known as strength, or pressure.
- Depth, or level at which the pulse prevails.
- Width, or breadth, also known as volume.
- Definition, also known as contour.
- Quality of Expansion, or rise / systole / pulsation.
- Quality of Interlude between Pulsations.
- Rhythm or Gait.
- Regularity
- Tension

The speed of the pulse is the frequency of its pulsations, measured in beats per minute. A normal or moderate speed is about 70 Beats per Minute (BPM); slow is under 70 BPM, to 60, or even below. A fast pulse is 80 BPM or higher. Basically, a fast pulse is indicative of excess heat or physical activity. The heat can be from an infection, inflammation or fever, which is often systemic. Exercise and digesting food also speed up the pulse.

Conversely, a slow pulse indicates coldness or hypoactivity. Those of a cold, Phlegmatic temperament also tend to have slow, deep pulses. However, those who are exceptionally fit, with aerobically trained and hyper efficient hearts can also have a slow pulse.

The force of the pulse most obviously indicates the strength of the Vital Force, and the overall vitality and energy level of the organism. The stronger the pulse, the more energy and vitality there is; the weaker the pulse, the weaker and more devitalized the body is.

A pulse that is extremely forceful and feels like it's bursting at the seams is not healthy, however; it indicates a condition of congestion or excess. A healthy pulse will also have all the organ pulses of equal, balanced, moderate strength; any undue force in an organ pulse indicates excess or congestion, whereas any undue weakness indicates emptiness or deficiency in that organ.

Depth refers to the level at which the pulse is felt. There are three basic levels, or depths, at which the pulse can be felt:

- Superficial: right below the skin, with light or no pressure.

- Moderate: middle depth, in between superficial and deep.

- Deep: felt with heavy pressure, right above the bone.

In taking the organ pulses, the pulses of the visceral organs, or related vessels, are felt at the Superficial level. The pulses of the deeper noble and principal organs are felt on the deep level.

In addition, there are certain commonly seen pulse types, or qualities, concerning depth that has clinical significance:

A Superficial Pulse, also known as a Floating Pulse, is one that is felt only or primarily at the Superficial level, fading or weakening effectively under deeper pressure. It generally indicates a superficial pathogen or dystemper, like the common cold. A superficial rapid pulse indicates exogenous heat, whereas a superficial slow or constricted pulse indicates exogenous cold.

A deep Pulse, which is felt only at the Deep level, can indicate two things: disharmonies of the deeper noble and principal organs; or excessive interior cold depress the pulse. A pulse that lacks sufficient heat will often lack sufficient vitality and exuberance to rise to the higher levels.

A Prominent Pulse is one that is felt most prominently at the Superficial level, but which also has good underlying strength and vitality at the other levels as well. It generally indicates abundant vitality and exuberance, and, in extreme cases, an excessively exuberant state of hyperexcitation.

A Rootless Pulse is one that is felt only at the Superficial and Moderate levels, but disappears at the Deep level, having no "root". It generally indicates a weakness or deficiency in the deep noble and principal organs, especially the kidneys.

The healthy pulse, in terms of depth, is felt most strongly at the middle depth or Moderate level, but also at the Superficial and Deep levels as well.

Width refers to the volume or breadth of the pulse. Is the pulse fat or skinny? Does it feel like a fine thread or a thick rope? A thin or skinny pulse is usually called a Thready Pulse, whereas a fat, broad pulse is usually called a Full Pulse. Most obviously and directly, a Full Pulse is associated with conditions of fullness, excess or superfluity; conversely, a Thready Pulse is associated with conditions of emptiness, or deficiency: The thinner the pulse, the greater the deficiency; the thicker the pulse, the greater the fullness or excess. The healthy pulse is moderate in width or breadth.

Definition refers to the clarity of the pulse's contour, or outline. Basically, conditions of dryness create a very clear, stark outline of the pulse. Conditions of moisture or wetness create a softness of pulse boundaries.

Closely related to this quality of definition is the continuum of hard versus soft, with hardness indicating dryness, and softness indicating moisture. Somtimes the hardness or softness of the artery walls can be felt, apparent and separate from the blood and other humors flowing through the artery. Atherosclerotic changes can often be felt in hard artery walls.

A Soggy Pulse has a special kind of softness that feels like an excessively soft and soggy overcooked noodle. It indicates a generalized lack of tone and consolidation of the Vital Force, and conditions of excess moisture and devitalization prevailing in the digestive system and Natural Faculty.

The healthy pulse should be adequately crisp and defined, but also have some softness.

Quality of Expansion refers to the quality of the rise, or pulsation of the artery. Aside from the pulsation's force, which has already been discussed, how long does the pulsation, or beat, last? How does it rise, and how does it fall? Are both the rising and the falling discrete and perceptible? Does one predominate over the other? The quality of the expansion or pulsation is a key factor in determining pulse gait.

The quality of interlude between pulsations is also an important factor to consider. How long is the gap between pulsations, relative to the duration of the pulsations themselves? Can the pulse still be felt, and maintain some perceptible level of pressure and contour between pulsations, or does it seem to disappear altogether? A pulse that is too weak or scattered in between pulsations can indicate systemic devitalization and insufficient consolidation of the Vital Force.

Rhythm or Gait is the overall characterization of the pulse, its particular feel, rhythm. You could say that the pulse gait is a synthesis of all the preceding factors. Pulse gaits are often described in terms of natural phenomena, like waves breaking on a beach. Or, pulse gaits can be likened to the movement of certain animals, like a leaping gazelle or crawling ants. Some common pulse gaits will be covered later.

Regularity is an important factor in the pulse, as irregularities can point to weaknesses or dysfunctions of the heart, whose contractions generate the pulse. Many of these heart weaknesses can be chronic or relatively mild in nature, and don't necessarily indicate an imminent acute cardiac crisis or major arrhythmia. However, a weak heart is indicated, which should be strengthened and supported with the right herbal tonics.

There are different types and degrees of irregularities in the pulse, with varying levels of seriousness and severity. Irregularities in the pulse can manifest in three basic forms, or aspects: in strength, or force; in speed or rhythm; and in skipped or missed beats. Of these three, the last is the most serious and the first the least.

Do the irregularities follow a regular, predictable pattern, or do they happen at random? Of course, irregular or random irregularities are more serious than regular ones. And yet another dimension to consider is: How frequently do the irregularities occur? Obviously, the more frequently irregularities occur, the more serious the condition. And so, the most serious type of irregularity is one of frequent, randomly occurring missed beats; regularly occurring or less frequent missed beats would be preferable.

Irregularity of pulse force usually consists of occasional or alternating weak beats interspersed amongst normal ones. Irregularity of speed or rhythm consists of periodic slowdowns and speedups of the pulse rate, or occasional hesitant or hasty beats. Episodes of a Racing Pulse are commonly associated with heart palpitations.

Pulse tension refers to the relative degree of tautness or laxness in the pulse. The healthy pulse should have sufficient relaxation and suppleness without being too lax. Excessive tension in the pulse is more problematic than excessive laxness.

A Tense or Wiry Pulse, also called a Twisted or Cordlike Pulse in Persian Medicine, feels like a taut string. It is associated either with chronic pain or emotional / psychosomatic stress and tension; or, it indicates Melancholic conditions of liver congestion and stagnation, portal hypertension, or gastrointestinal colic. A Tense Pulse can also indicate arterial hypertension.

Pulse length is closely associated with pulse tension, because a tense pulse is often long. If the pulse is long, but also supple and relaxed, however, this is not particularly pathological or abnormal.

A Short Pulse is usually felt in one position only, which is usually, but not always, the Median position. If the pulse is detectable at all, it can usually be felt in the Median position. A Short Pulse denotes a deficiency of the Vital Force.

Pulse and Temperament

The Four Basic Qualities are detectable in the basic parameters of the pulse. By mixing and matching these pulse parameters, you obtain the pulses for the compound temperaments.

The pulses indicative of the four compound temperaments is not necessarily constitutional in nature. They do, however, indicate conditions of compound temperament currently prevailing in the body.

A hot temperament is primarily indicated by a rapid pulse. Pulses that are prominent, forceful or bounding also tend to be hot in that they are energetic and exuberant in nature. Somtimes, the heat can even be felt directly, as when the artery itself feels hot or Hot to the touch.

A cold temperament is primarily indicated by a slow pulse, especially if the cold is endogenous or chronic. Chronic or endogenous cold can also sink the pulse, making it deep. A weak pulse can also be a sign of cold, since it indicates a lack of energy. Acute or exogenous cold, as in catching a cold or a chill, can constrict the pulse; the quality of constriction is something akin to tension, but not quite. A longstanding cold dystemper can also produce a tense pulse.

A wet temperament, or excessive moisture, is primarily indicated by a soft or soggy pulse. A full pulse could also possibly be classified as wet or moist, since it indicates and excess, abundance or superfluity of blood and/or other humors.

A slippery pulse is another distinctive pulse type, or gait, that's usually associated with excess dampness and phlegm. It's found in pregnant women, who need increased amounts of the moist, flourishing Phlegmatic and Sanguine humors to nourish their growing fetus. The pulsations of a slippery pulse aren't felt pushing vertically against the fingers as much as they are felt slithering by laterally; when you try to pin it down, it rolls out from under your fingers like pearls in a porcelain bowl.

A dry temperament is indicated primarily by a pulse that is clearly defined, crisp and hard, or firm. Somtimes, the hardness or firmness can be felt in the artery wall, rather than in its contents. A thin pulse is also dry in temperament, since it denotes a lack or deficiency of moist flourishing humors; it's even dryer if it is also clearly defined.

Roughness is another quality commonly found in dry pulses, and is contrary to the smoothness of the slippery pulse. A choppy pulse is rough and abrupt, and is often associated with a Dry temperament. If a choppy pulse should also be thin, it denotes a deficiency of blood and the Radical Moisture. Otherwise, it indicates a systemic stagnation of blood.

As with heat, the relative moisture level of the artery can Somtimes be felt directly. The artery of a wet pulse will often feel moist or clammy.

By mixing and matching some of these basic pulse parameters, you can obtain composite pulses characteristic of the four compound temperaments, as follows:

Sanguine (Hot and moist): moderate speed to slightly rapid, and moderately soft and relaxed, with good vitality.

Choleric (Hot and dry): rapid, forceful and clearly defined.

Melancholic (Cold and dry): slow or weak, tense or constricted, thin and clearly defined.

Phlegmatic (Cold and wet): deep, slow and soft.

Other Important Pulse Gaits

There are several other pulse gaits that are distinctive and important. I will discuss a few of them here.

An Empty Pulse is big in width, but lacks strength or forcefulness; it is also felt superficially, and tends to be slower than normal. It denotes a deficiency of blood and the Vital Force.

A Hollow Pulse also feels empty; it feels hollow. It is usually seen after an extreme loss of blood, which can no longer adequately fill the artery.

A Flooding Pulse surges up like a wave breaking upon the shore, quite big and strong, but falls with considerably less force. It denotes that heat has injured the Phlegmatic humor, serous fluids and Radical Moisture.

APersian Medicine pulse that is similar is the Waving Pulse, which also has a wavelike quality. However, the waves are weak, irregular in largeness, rhythm and degree of rise, and often break one upon the other. A weakness of the Vital Force is usually the cause; the Waving Pulse can also indicate that a healing crisis, either by perspiration or diarrhea, is imminent.

A Disappearing Pulse is one that rises up clearly and then disappears after reaching the top of the pulsation; its rises are felt, but its falls are absent. The outlines of this pulse can also be a little rough and diffuse. It indicates a critical deficiency of both the blood and the Vital Force, and is usually seen in extreme exhaustion, or after feats of severe physical exertion.

Another pulse is the Gazelle Pulse, which is like the leap of a gazelle - hopping up quickly, obtaining a level plateau, then abruptly rising and trailing off at the end. A distinctive feature of this pulse is that the next beat, or gazelle leap, starts before the previous one is finished. Its cause is the heat associated with fever; it can also indicate pericarditis.

A Hurried Pulse is one that is both rapid and intermittent, occasionally skipping beats at irregular intervals. It indicates that heat is agitating both the blood and Vital Force.

A Minute Pulse is both weak in force, thin in width, and nebulous in its contour, being indistinct and barely perceptible. It indicates extreme weakness, devitalization and deficiency.

A Scattered Pulse is like an Empty Pulse because it is big or wide, superficial and weak. However, its contour is fuzzy, scattered and diffuse, and it falls or recedes much more strongly than it rises. It indicates extreme adrenal exhaustion.

An Ant-like or Formicant Pulse feels like a line or ants crawling up a tree, and is extremely feeble, scattered and diffuse. *Hakim Chishti* says that it indicates a weakness of peristaltic action.

Urine diagnosis

The art of urine diagnosis, or uroscopy, is an important part of Persian Medicine. Avicenna devotes considerable space to it in his Canon of Medicine.

The medical treatises of Avicenna became the basis for medical practice in Europe in the high middle Ages, and an important part of this was uroscopy, or urine diagnosis. So important was uroscopy as a diagnostic method that taking a sample of one's morning urine before going to see the doctor was almost obligatory.

Nowadays, taking a urine sample is still done for some things, but the modern doctor uses microscopes, test strips, and all manner of sophisticated biochemical tests to analyze the urine sample. Methods of urine analysis were much simpler, utilizing observation and the senses in simple tests.

The Clinical Significance of the Urine

As long as there is life, there is pepsis, or digestion and metabolism. Elimination, or the excretion of unusable wastes, is the final stage of pepsis; all metabolic processes generate waste.

The wastes generated by the metabolic processes of the body can tell the physician a lot about these processes. And so it is with urine, which is the principal liquid waste of the body; the urine provides the physician with a window into the inner metabolic processes of the organism.

The wastes of the First Digestion are excreted via the stool. But the wastes from the Second through Fourth stages of digestion, from the initial coction and generation of the humors in the liver until their final assimilation and transmutation into living tissue, are excreted mainly via the urine.

Besides excreting liquid wastes, the kidneys, through the production and discharge of urine, also work to balance the humors and chemistry of the bloodstream. Any excesses or superfluities are thrown off, while that which is in short supply is conserved. But what is most apparent and visible in the urine are those superfluities which are being eliminated.

Although careful inspection of the urine will yield much information about many metabolic processes of the body, the urine most directly indicates the state of the liver and the condition of the genitourinary organs and their passages and vessels.

Technique of Urine Diagnosis

To obtain accurate and reliable results from urine diagnosis, it's important that the urine sample be collected and prepared in the right way. And here's how it's done:

The urine to be collected for the urine sample is to be that of the morning's first urine, unless instructed otherwise by the physician. And the urine to be collected in the urine jar or flask is to be a mid-stream catch, avoiding the initial flow as well as the final portion. The urine jar or container should preferably be of clear glass or crystal, freshly washed, cleaned and dried, both inside and out. For accurate color observation, the glass should be free from any undue coloring. Glass is preferable to plastic, since it's more chemically inert.

The urine collected in the jar should be collected upon arising, before one has had anything to eat or drink. In particular, within the previous day or two, one should refrain from eating foods that might unduly color the urine, such as saffron (yellow-orange) or beets (red). Also, avoid sex before taking the urine sample, as well as any activities or conditions that would effectively alter the humoral balance or metabolism from its usual state, such as fasting, sleeplessness or purgatives.

Of course, a label with one's name on it should be affixed to the lid of the jar, as identification for the physician. The physician should not inspect the urine sample right after it has been collected, but should wait a while, so any sediment that might be present can form and settle out; an hour or so after the initial collection is ideal. Six hours or more, according to Avicenna, is too long.

Before the urine sample is inspected by the physician, the patient should take care to keep it away from extremes of heat, coldness, direct sunlight, or other undue exposure to the elements. These can damage or alter the urine sample.

Basic Parameters of Urine Diagnosis

The physician inspects the urine for the following basic parameters:

- Color
- Consistency - degree of thickness or thinness; viscosity
- Clarity - degree of clearness or turbidity (cloudiness)
- Sediment - presence or absence, and type of sediment
- Foam - characteristics of foam formed either initially, or when shaken vigorously

▪ Odor - either absence of odor or the presence of strong, offensive or unusual odors

In addition to the above six parameters, which can be observed in the urine sample directly, the physician usually makes inquiries as to the patient's urinary habits. These inquiries concern the following:

▪ Urinary frequency and volume - used to ascertain whether the patient suffers from oliguria (deficient urination) or polyuria (excessive urination); or, if his/her urinary output is moderate. Somtimes, the physician will ask the patient to collect all the urine voided within a 24-hour period in order to get a more accurate assessment of total daily urine output. A normal or average daily urine output is 1500 ml.
▪ Frequent, urgent, and/or painful urination - these are the cardinal signs of a urinary tract infection.
▪ Nocturia or getting up at night to urinate - a cardinal sign of chronic urinary weakness or debility.
▪ Dribbling, retention or incomplete voiding of urine - besides indicating the possible presence of obstructing urinary stones, sand in both sexes, these signs, plus frequent or urgent urination, are usually indicative of an enlarged prostate in mature or elderly men.

Basic Parameters of Urine and Temperament

The first two of the six basic urine parameters listed previously concern the Four Basic Qualities and basic parameters of temperament. Color most pertains to the primary or active polarity of Hot / Cold. Consistency most pertains to the secondary or passive polarity of dry / wet.

The basic color continuum starts with white or colorless at the cold end of the scale, and moves through increasingly darker shades of yellow until a very dark yellow is arrived at at the hot end. And so:

-Cold means white, or colorless

-Hot means dark yellow

-Moderate means straw colored or citron yellow.

-With urine consistency, the basic continuum is quite simple:

-Dry means thin or light, watery urine

-Wet means thick or dense, heavy urine

-Moderate means neither too thick nor too thin.

And so, the four compound temperaments, or the Four Temperaments, typically produce the following basic types of urine:

Sanguine (Hot and moist): bright yellow, showing moderate heat; and slightly thick, showing moderate moisture.

Choleric (Hot and dry): dark yellow, showing extreme heat; and thin, showing dryness. Urine may also be concentrated and scanty due to dryness.

Melancholic (Cold and Dry): white, or colorless, showing coldness; and thin, showing dryness.

Phlegmatic (Cold and Wet): white or colorless, showing coldness; and thick, showing wetness.

In addition, there's the all-important dimension of urine volume. White or colorless urine indicates coldness prevailing in the organism, and a deficiency of the Metabolic Heat, which isn't ripening sufficient uric acid and other toxins for elimination. It is with white or colorless urine that abnormalities or extremes of urine volume most commonly occur.

With colorless scanty urine, a deficient Metabolic Heat is getting flooded or drowned out by excessive Water. Deficient urine output means undue retention of water and fluids within the body. The basic temperament of this condition is Phlegmatic; the urine is usually thick.

With colorless abundant urine, or polyuria, a deficient Metabolic Heat is unable to reabsorb, re-circulate, and re-metabolize fluids back into the organism. Excessive urine output means a deficiency of fluids remaining in the body, and is therefore dry and Melancholic in temperament. This urine picture is often associated with aesthenic or wasting conditions. Diabetes insipidus, or the passing of large amounts of watery, tasteless, insipid urine, also fits this picture.

Urine Color

Basically, the level of color present in the urine indicates the level of Metabolic Heat that the kidneys have at their disposal to ripen and eliminate uric acid and other wastes and superfluous humors from the body.

White or colorless urine generally indicates a Cold temperament prevailing in the organism; there is insufficient metabolic heat to adequately ripen the toxins and other wastes for elimination. Besides coldness, colorless, watery urine can also be due to excessive fluid consumption, and consequently fluid elimination, which is diluting the urine; if such is the case, the volume of urine being passed will usually be copious.

The basic normal color of urine, if it is to have color, is various shades of yellow. This typical yellow color we now know to be due primarily to the presence of uric acid, but it was considered to be a manifestation of the action of the Metabolic Heat; the greater the heat, the darker the shade of yellow. Persian Medicine considers the yellowness of the urine to be a byproduct or waste product, of the hot, bilious humor in the liver.

Avicenna, in the Canon of Medicine, describes the various possible shades of yellow as: straw yellow, citron yellow, reddish yellow, orange-yellow, flame yellow; saffron yellow, also called perfect yellow; and saffron colored, or bright red.

Straw yellow and citron yellow, Avicenna states, denote a balanced, normal heat level and an equable temperament. Lighter shades of yellow would be colder in temperament.

The darker saffron and flame shades of yellow denote a hotter, bilious temperament. This is particularly true of acute hot natured diseases. With extreme heat, the urine can even be brownish in color. Insufficient fluids can also concentrate the urine and turn it a darker color. And then, bright yellow colored urine can also be due to the consumption of vitamin supplements.

Generally, tints or shades of urine other than yellow denote more abnormal, morbid conditions. Often, the tint of the urine will indicate the nature of the morbid humor or superfluity.

Obviously, urine tinted red usually indicates the presence of blood, or hematuria; most commonly, there is bleeding in the bladder, kidneys or urinary tract. Some foods, like saffron or beets, may color the urine red.

Brown urine is usually a very concentrated form of yellow, denoting an extremely hot or bilious temperament. Brown urine is usually associated with biliousness, jaundice, or the abnormal charring of bile. The heat level is even greater if the urine burns when being excreted.

Urine which is the color of fresh meat washings is a grave sign. It can indicate an excess or superfluity of blood, but most often, it indicates a weakness or unbalanced, bad temperament of the liver; in such states, there is also a weakness of pepsis, or digestion, and a dispersion of vitality.

Green urine generally indicates a lack of Innate Heat, and an insufficient combustion or coction of the humors. A bright rainbow green is usually indicative of poisoning, and is particularly serious if no sediment is present. A green resembling bronze rust or patina indicates a total extinguishing of the Innate Heat, and is usually terminal.

Black, dark brown, gray or ashen shades of urine are generally associated with black bile. A greenish black denotes the presence of normal black bile. A brownish black is associated with Sanguineous forms of black bile. Black urine that is very dark is a grave sign; it can either indicate a high level of charring, or oxidation; great interior cold; impending death; or a great catharsis of superfluous black bile.

The passing of dark or abnormal shades of urine can be a good sign if it occurs in acute diseases, especially at the time of the crisis, which is a catharsis, or cleansing of morbid matter from the body. If seen at the beginning or at the end of an acute illness, however, it is generally an unfavorable sign. Dark urine passed in the elderly or in the chronically ill, does not inform well, and often indicates a great destruction of the internal organs and tissues.

Urine Consistency, Viscosity or Texture

Determining urine thickness or viscosity isn't as simple or straightforward as observing its color. Nevertheless, there are a number of ways this can be done.

The most obvious and direct way to test for urine viscosity is to rub a little bit of the sample between your thumb and forefinger to see how it feels.

Avicenna mainly compares thick urine with a subtle kind of inconsistency or turbidity. When a specimen of thick, clear urine is held at a distance, it will appear to be perfectly clear, but when carefully examined up close, fine lines or markings will become visible in it. Thin clear urine, on the other hand, will appear perfectly clear and uniform whether examined up close or from afar.

Another way to test for urine viscosity is to shake the sample vigorously and see what kind of froth or foam appears on its surface. The foam formed in thin urine will consist of smaller, finer bubbles, which will burst or dissolve more quickly; thick urine will form larger bubbles, which will linger for a long time before bursting or subsiding.

Another way to test for urine viscosity is the oil drop test. Take a dropper filled with Olive oil and drop a drop into the urine sample. The greater the urine viscosity, the less that oil drop will disperse; conversely, the thinner the viscosity, the more the oil drops will disperse.

In extremely thick urine, the oil drop will not disperse at all, remaining suspended just below the surface like a round pearl. Such thick, clear urine shows that the kidneys are secreting a lot of superfluous thick phlegm into the urine. Such urine is Phlegmatic in temperament, and is often seen in Phlegmatic diseases like epilepsy or diabetes.

In extremely thin urine, the oil drop will disperse widely, creating an extremely fine, iridescent film on the urine's surface. Thin urine denotes conditions of Dry temperament prevailing in the organism, and is often seen in asthenic, wasting conditions and deficiency states. Thin urine is generally dry and Melancholic in temperament, especially if also white or colorless.

Urine Clarity versus Turbidity

Is the urine clear, or is it cloudy, or turbid? Obviously, clear urine is healthier, and preferable to cloudy urine.

There are basically two major phases of pepsis, or the process of digestion and metabolism, which are reflected in the urine:

The first phase of pepsis is called coction, which starts with the initial digestion of food into chyle in the GI tract, and culminates in the liver, with the coction, or generation of the Four Humors. This phase of pepsis is reflected mainly in the basic color and texture of the urine.

The second phase of pepsis is called maturation, which starts with the Four Humors after they are generated in the liver, and culminates with their formation, or maturation, into living tissue. Errors, imbalances and defects in this maturation process are seen mainly in the turbidity and sediment that forms in the urine.

Cloudy urine also indicates interior cold and a lack of vitality, which is impeding the maturation process. Since the cloudiness is usually white in color, the unripened humors are usually of a cold, Phlegmatic nature and temperament.

According to Persian Medicine, a cloudiness or smokiness that lingers right above the bottom of the urine sample indicates that the illness will be prolonged. If this condition of the urine persists throughout the course of the illness, it could indicate impending death. Urine that's clear when passed, but then becomes cloudy shows that the Metabolic Heat is having a harder time maturing the humors then if the urine is cloudy when passed, but soon clears.

Cloudy urine usually indicates the presence of unripen Phlegmatic humors. Cloudy or milky white urine with an offensive odor indicates the presence of pus, which is usually due to a ruptured abscess in the urinary tract.

Cloudiness in the urine usually is due to the presence of superfine particles that are in a state of colloidal suspension. Bigger, heavier particles tend to separate out as sediment.

Urine Sediment

There are many types of sediment that can be found in the urine, of various colors and textures. Generally, the quicker the sediment separates out, and the more completely it does so, the better the sign, or prognosis. Quicker and cleaner settling sediment shows that the morbid matter was closer to being properly matured and ripened at the time of urination.

Sediments are usually white, but can also be of some other color, like red, yellow, dusky or black. Sediment can also either be smooth in texture or rough. The daily passage of sediment in the urine is worse than the occasional passage of sediment, as it indicates that new unripened residues build up before old ones can be completely eliminated; usually, the texture of such daily sediment is not uniform or smooth.

The occasional passage of smooth white sediment in the urine isn't necessarily a bad thing, and can be noted in the urine of healthy persons as well. Avicenna notes that sediment is much more common in patients who are sedentary and overweight than in those who are lean and active. The precipitation of sediment in the urine is preferable to turbidity that doesn't settle or precipitate, and shows better maturation of the superfluous matter.

White is generally the best color for sediment, and after that, a reddish tint. Then comes yellow or dusky colored sediment. A black residue, or sediment, can be due either to intense heat or to intense cold. If the sediment is first dusky, then turns black it is due to cold; if first yellow, then black, it is due to heat. Rough sediment is usually due to flatulence, or the presence of thick, crude, undigested air or gases in the urine.

The most serious and abnormal kinds of sediment are various kinds of flaky sediment, which modern medicine calls casts. These flakes can also often resemble bran. Most often, these flakes are from the destruction of tissue, usually from erosion or degeneration of the mucous membranes and passages of the bladder and urinary tract, Generally, the larger the flakes, or casts, the more serious the condition. Flaky sediment that looks brown like fish scales is a particularly bad sign. Red flakes can be due to particles of clotted blood.

Sand or gravel in the urine will often cause problems and difficulties in voiding the urine. This is usually due to urinary stones forming in the kidneys or bladder.

Urine Foam

The degree of foam or froth present in the urine generally indicates the amount of dissolved gas present in the urine when it's passed. Persons who pass very foamy urine generally suffer from digestive gas, bloating and flatulence. A dark or orange colored froth denotes jaundice. If the bubbles are large, and their bursting or resolution slow, this denotes, besides the presence of gas, that the urine is thick, sticky or viscid. Thin, light urine produces small bubbles that burst or resolve rather quickly. If urine with small, fine bubbles persists for an extended time in kidney diseases, the disease will not be resolved quickly.

If the urine doesn't have much foam when it comes out, then gas is not an issue. However, shaking the urine sample vigorously and noting what kind of bubbles and foam are produced is one way of testing the urine for its overall thickness, stickiness and viscosity level.

Urine Odor

When normal urine is passed, it has a characteristic odor. However, if its odor should be strong, offensive, or otherwise strange or unusual, this indicates imbalance and pathology.

Normal urine should have a readily apparent, characteristic odor. Urine with absolutely no odor shows abnormal coldness and a deficiency of the Metabolic Heat.

An offensive odor, if the urine should be milky and white, is usually due to pus. If foul smelling urine is passed with good signs of maturation, it generally indicates scabies or ulcerations of the urinary organs. If foul smelling urine with poor or no signs of maturation is passed, the foul odor is due to raw, unripen humors, or to putrefaction.

Urine with a sweetish odor points to a predominance of blood, or a Sanguine condition. Everyone is familiar with the sweet, fruity smell of urine in diabetes.

Urine with a foul odor generally indicates the predominance of yellow bile. Urine with a foul and sour odor indicates a predominance of black bile.

The passage of foul or abnormal smelling urine need not be a cause for alarm, and often happens in healthy persons as well as sick ones. When fasting, or when undergoing a healing crisis or catharsis, foul smelling urine indicates the release of toxins. If passage of such urine should bring the healthy person a feeling of relief, and of increased health and wellbeing, it is a good sign that a beneficial catharsis has taken place.

Final Thoughts on Urine Volume

Although you could say that the average normal daily urine volume is about 1500 ml, what constitutes normal, healthy urine function is all relative to the volume of fluids consumed. Drink more, urinate more; drink less, urinate less.

Where the real abnormalities come in is if someone drinks a lot, yet urinates relatively little; this is oliguria. Conversely, polyuria can be defined as someone who drinks moderately or very little, but nevertheless urinates a lot. Normal versus abnormal urinary function and output is always defined as relative to the fluid volume consumed. Difficulties passing urine, dribbling it drop by drop or obstructions to the urinary flow are also causes for concern. Particularly if urine of a dark, abnormal color or a strong odor, or other abnormalities has difficulties being passed, it is a bad sign; for a good catharsis, such urine should be passed freely. Dribbling urine, involuntary urination, and urinary incontinence are signs of neuromuscular degeneration in the urinary organs. Urination that is too frequent, as well as nocturia, is signs of urinary debility.

Diagnosis from the stool

In Persian Medicine, diagnosis can also be done by examining the stool. Usually, general questions about the patient's stool and bowel habits are asked in the medical history, but when actual examination is needed, the physician will ask the patient to bring a stool sample in for inspection.

Both the urine and the stool can be examined to yield valuable diagnostic information, but, examining samples of the patient's urine is done more frequently than examining the stool. When methods of simple visual examination of the stool are insufficient, the contemporary practitioner of Persian Medicine will have modern lab tests of the stool for things like ova and parasites, or occult blood, done.

The patient is asked to collect a sample of his/her stool in a small glass jar or plastic container. The container must be clean, and have a tight, securely fitting lid. Besides being examined visually, the sample is also smelled for odor and probed with an instrument to examine its basic hardness, consistency and texture as well as checking it for the presence of any undigested food or foreign matter.

The Physiology of Defecation

The stool is the principal waste product of the First Digestion, which occurs in the gastrointestinal tract. After the chyle, or creamy juice essence of the food, is extracted and absorbed in the intestinal tract, the unusable waste that remains forms the stool. And so, examination of the stool yields the most information about the nature, temperament and overall quality of the initial First Digestion of food and drink in the GI tract.

In its trip down the GI tract on its way to becoming the stool, the semi-liquefied food juices are acted on by the Four Humors, which are products of the Second Digestion, which happens in the liver. Each one of these humors has its own inherent force, or Administrative Virtue, which determines how it acts upon the semi-liquefied food juices in the formation and expulsion of the stool. For normal, healthy defecation, all the Four Humors must be working harmoniously together in the right balance or proportion.

Blood, or the Sanguine humor, has an Attractive force, or virtue. Blood running through the fine capillaries in the villi of the small intestine attracts, or draws in, nutrients from the chyle into itself, and is responsible for the initial absorption of raw nutrients, which are sent to the liver for processing into the Four Humors. Blood also carries the vital principles that power the functioning of the peristaltic muscles that send the food juices or bolus along on its way towards becoming the stool.

Phlegm, or the Phlegmatic humor, has an Expulsive force, or virtue. Phlegmatic secretions of the GI mucosa act as a lubricant, smoothing the peristaltic flow of the food juices or bolus along its way towards defecation. A sufficient quantity of fluids, or the Water element, must remain in the stool to give it the necessary softness that makes defecation possible. The normal, healthy stool is not purely solid, but rather semi-solid. If we don't adequately feed the Phlegmatic humor with sufficient fluids and juicy, moist fresh fruits and vegetables, we will get constipated, and find proper stool expulsion difficult.

Yellow bile, or the Choleric humor, has a Digestive force, or virtue. It is secreted by the liver and gall bladder directly into the duodenum and small intestine. Its main job there is to excrete, digest and absorb fats, but it's hot, sharp, mildly irritating quality also acts to stimulation peristaltic movement and the defecation reflex in the large intestine. This makes bile the body's own natural laxative. Normal healthy bile is what colors the stool a rich, dark brown; stools that are too light in color usually lack sufficient bile.

Black bile, or the Melancholic humor, has a Retentive force, or virtue. The action of black bile, with its drying quality and Retentive force, works to reabsorb vital fluids and solidify the stool in the large intestine. Black bile gives the stool the necessary solidity that enables it to be retained until the time is right for defecation. Excessive amounts of black bile, however, lead to excessive retention, or constipation.

Stool formation and defecation is the main function of the large intestine. Phlegm softens and lubricates the stool, favoring expulsion. Black bile condenses and solidifies the stool, favoring retention. Into this delicate balance steps yellow bile, this tips the scales in favor of defecation.

Stool Patterns of the Four Temperaments

Each of the Four Temperaments has typical stool patterns and bowel habits associated with it, according to the nature of its predominant humor. In addition, acquired conditions and disorders affecting the stool can be broadly differentiated according to the classical concepts of humor and temperament. For each of the Four Temperaments, I will first discuss the typical patterns and tendencies of the normal individual, and then

I will discuss some common acquired conditions and disorders pertaining to that humor and temperament.

Sanguine (Hot and Moist): Since Sanguine is considered to be the most equable and balanced of all the temperaments, its stool patterns and bowel habits are also generally the healthiest and desirable. The Sanguine stool has adequate, generous bulk; has the perfect balance between softness and firmness, and is well-formed; has a rich brown color, and no unpleasant odor.

Some say that, because blood is the predominant humor in the Sanguine temperament, that the Sanguine stool frequently has a reddish tint. But any presence of blood in the stool is abnormal and pathological. Bleeding from the colon and rectum will show up as red blood leeching out from the stool, and bleeding from higher up in the GI tract will often show up as tarry patches in the stools; or, the blood may be hidden, or occult. Certain foods, like beets, can also color the stool a bloody red.

Those of a Sanguine temperament have an addiction for overeating, eating rich food, and not getting adequate fiber. Food that is too nutrient dense and fiber poor will tend to stagnate, ferment and putrefy in the digestive tract and bowels. There will be abdominal bloating, sluggish bowels, constipation, foul smelling gas and flatulence, and stools that are soft, gummy and foul smelling. Putrefaction is basically a Sanguine condition of excess Hotth and moisture.

Medical recognition of the importance of fiber is nothing new. Thousand years ago, Avicenna praised the health benefits of fiber.

Phlegmatic (Cold and wet): The typical Phlegmatic stool is large, copious and soft, indicating the presence of excess phlegm and dampness. There is no strong or offensive odor. The texture of the normal Phlegmatic stool is smooth and moist.

Soft, sluggish Phlegmatic stools are often associated with a slow, deficient pepsis and a hypoactivity of the Metabolic Heat and digestive fire. If the stools should also be loose with pieces of undigested food in them, this indicates a serious case of dyspepsia.

Another common Phlegmatic type of stool is the mucoid stool; the stool will have visible streaks, or veins, of mucus running through it. Clumps or deposits of semisolid phlegm, or mucus, can accumulate in the intestines and digestive tract just like they can in the nose, throat and respiratory tract.

Phlegmatic loose stools or diarrhea will often occur in the early morning upon arising. This is the time of day when the Metabolic Heat is at its lowest.

Choleric (Hot and dry): Yellow bile, with its hot, sharp quality, has a laxative effect and provokes the defecation reflex. Since yellow bile is the dominant humor in those of a Choleric temperament, stools will tend to be soft, greasy or unctuous, and may often have a strong or foul odor. Intestinal transit time tends to be short, since the Metabolic Heat is very active in Choleric.

If there is an infection of the bowels, which is another Choleric condition of excess heat, the bowels will be agitated, and the diarrhea more urgent and severe. The more virulent the infection, the quicker and severe will be the diarrhea. In dysentery, not only will there be quick diarrhea, but blood may also be present in the stools. Ulcerative colitis will produce diarrhea mixed with blood and mucus.

If bile is congested in the liver and gall bladder and isn't flowing smoothly, there will often be constipation. The stools will be hard, dry and compact from the excess heat, and light in color, due to the deficiency of bile. In these cases, laxatives are needed to stimulation the flow of bile and remove blockages and obstructions to its flow.

Somtimes, both phlegm and bile are excessive, or aggravated. In these cases, the stools will be large and abundant, soft, slimy, smelly, and bright yellow. The stool will often burn the anus as its being passed. There may also be a sallow, jaundiced complexion, a sluggish digestion or indigestion, and generalized lethargy or malaise.

Abnormal forms of yellow bile will color the stools green. This usually indicates that the Innate Heat of pepsis, or digestion and metabolism, is low.

Melancholic (Cold and dry): Because of the Retentive virtue of black bile, the dominant humor in those of a Melancholic temperament, constipation is common. When the stools come out, they are usually small, hard, compact and dry, and may have a silvery gray sheen to them, which indicates the presence of black bile.

Melancholic also suffer from colicky digestive complaints, with lots of gas, distension and bloating. If a lot of gas is present in the stool, it will float in the toilet bowl. An even larger amount of gas, or flatulence, will honeycomb the stools, making them rough, irregular in shape, and spongy. Such stools are also called costive, and are a common stool type seen in Melancholic individuals, as well as those with excess wind and black bile in the bowels.

Irritable bowel is another common syndrome seen in Melancholic individuals, and is characterized by alternating constipation and diarrhea. Morbid charred or oxidized forms of black and yellow bile, which are irritating to the GI mucosa, are often associated with this condition.

If large amounts of black bile are passed in the stool, the stools will be blackish in color. This is generally not a good sign.

Basic Diagnostic Parameters of the Stool

There are certain basic parameters of the stool that the physician considers in making his assessment of the patient's condition. These are the stool's volume, color, consistency and odor.

Stool Volume should be commensurate with the amount of food and drink consumed. An abundant stool is one whose volume is excessive in relation to the quantity of food and drink consumed. A scanty stool is one whose volume is significantly less relative to the amount of food and drink consumed.

When the stool is copious, there are basically two things that could be going on. The first possibility is that the digestive system and Natural Faculty aren't efficiently extracting all the nutritive essences from the food and drink consumed. This is generally called an assimilation disorder, and is usually associated with a weak pepsis and digestive fire. Certain food allergies or sensitivities to things like gluten can also create stools like this.

The second possibility is that the organism is using the stool to discharge excessive or superfluous humors that have accumulated. This is often something that is out of the ordinary, and the patient may make a remark about it. Under the right conditions, wastes that have been held within the body and in the bowels may be discharged, or released.

If there is an inadequate digestion and absorption of nutrients, the patient will be tired and run-down, especially after passing the stool. If excessive or superfluous humors are being discharged, defecation should bring relief and an enhanced sense of wellbeing.

If the stool is scanty, the usual problem is that the stools aren't being completely evacuated, and excess fecal matter is being retained in the cecum and colon. Chronically retained fecal matter may become impacted, and retained wastes may back up all the way into the small intestine, causing colic, gas and reflux symptoms in the middle and upper digestive tract.

Persian Medicine stresses the importance of proper intestinal waste management, and keeping the bowels clean and functioning properly. Constipation is called the Mother of All Diseases. The bowels of the human body can be compared to the roots of a tree; if the colon is congested and toxic, it's like the roots of the body are being poisoned, which will poison the whole organism.

If the stools are copious, they are also usually soft; such is the nature of the moist, flourishing humors of the organism. If the stools are scanty, they are usually, but not always, hard, dry and compacted. Wetness feeds and flourishes, dryness withers and shrinks.

If the stools are soft and loose but also scanty, there are also usually colicky symptoms involved. Such is often the case in irritable bowel, intestinal infections and parasites. In dysentery, there can be marked tenesmus, or a desire and urge to evacuate the bowels which is unproductive, in addition to frequent loose stools and diarrhea.

Stool Color should be, normally, a rich, deep brown. This indicates that the bile is flowing smoothly. If the bile is not flowing smoothly, the stools will be a light brown, yellowish or pale colored. If there is excessive phlegm and dampness as well as an aggravation of bile, the stools will be a bright yellow. Greenish stools indicate a deficient Innate Heat of pepsis and digestion. Stools with a reddish tint indicate the possible presence of blood. Black bile will color the stools a steely gray, or make them blackish in color. Back, tarry stools can indicate bleeding higher up in the GI tract. Reddish stools are often passed at the crisis point of a disease.

Stool Consistency should be semisolid - firm, but not hard, and well-formed. Basically, soft or loose stools are Wet in temperament, whereas hard, compact stools are Dry.

Soft or loose stools, if they do not foul smell, generally indicate a deficient pepsis and metabolic heat that don't concoct or ripen the stool and reabsorb excess fluids adequately. If the stools are soft and slimy, this usually indicates excess phlegm.

Soft or loose stools that do have a foul odor are usually due to aggravated bile and excess heat and choler. Signs and symptoms of urgency or irritable bowel may also be present.

Porous, costive or irregularly shaped stools are usually due to the presence of excess wind - flatulence, or gas. Such stools will usually float in the toilet bowl.

Stool Odor in the normal stool should not be totally absent; a healthy stool should have a characteristic musky odor. Odors in excess of this, or strange and unusual odors, are definitely abnormal. Most cases of a foul-smelling stool are due either to fermentation or putrefaction in the intestines, or to aggravated yellow bile. A rotten odor of the stool is often indicative of an imbalance of intestinal flora.

Principles of treatment

Introduction to therapeutics in Persian Medicine

Healing with Contraries

In Persian Medicine, the usual way of treating disease is through the use of medicines and treatments that are contrary in nature to that of the disease or disorder. Avicenna explains:

Diseases which arise from repletion are cured by depletion; and those which arise from depletion are cured by repletion; and in general, diseases are cured by their contraries.

Excesses must be drained or purged; deficiencies must be supplemented by what is missing. Fevers must be cooled down; chills must be dispelled with heat and Hot. Roughness and dryness must be smoothed and moistened. Excess wetness and moisture must be dried up and dispersed. Blockages and obstructions must also be dispersed.

In supplementing deficiencies, we must seek out and use medicines and treatments that will provide the desired quality or nutritional factor that is lacking. The principle here is:

- In correcting imbalances, we must seek out and use medicines and treatments that are contrary in nature to that of the imbalance. The principle here is: Opposites balance. Furthermore, while being contrary in quality, medicines or treatments for correcting imbalances must be similar in degree to the severity of the imbalance; otherwise, we run the risk of either underdoing the correction or leaving some of the original imbalance behind, or of overdoing the correction and creating a new imbalance that is contrary in nature to the first. We need just the right touch.

In removing or purging excesses, congestions and obstructions, we must know and make our treatment appropriate to three factors:

1) What is in excess, causing the congestion and obstruction;

2) Where in the body the excess, congestion or obstruction is;

3) How much, or how severe, is the congestion or obstruction.

We must use medicines and treatments that specifically address all three of these above factors if we are going to be successful:

You wouldn't use a medicine to purge phlegm if blood or bile was the congesting or obstructing factor.

You wouldn't use a medicine to purge the head if it was the bowels that suffered from excess or congestion;

In all cases, the medicine or treatment must be appropriate and well-matched to the degree or severity of the disorder.

Using these measures of kind, part and degree, the physician or therapist works to undo or reverse the damage that the disease process has created, to lead the patient back from a state of disorder, or disease, to one of order, or health.

▪ If the patient is clearly suffering from a deficiency disorder, then we must obviously supplement and build. Conversely, if a patient is clearly suffering from plethora and excess, we should purge, or cleanse the offending matter.

But many patients are suffering from a little of both - excess and deficiency. Then, what do you do?

In these cases, Persian Medicine gives initial preference to cleansing.

"In bodies not properly cleansed, the more you nourish, the more you injure."

In bodies whose vital channels have become clogged with toxic and morbid matter, these same vessels cannot carry nutrients to the tissues for proper assimilation. So, these nutrients just wind up stagnating and putrefying, injuring us and making us sick.

A couple of analogies here would make things clearer: A full cup cannot hold any more water; it must first be emptied to receive more.

The cleansing can be mild and gentle; it need not be radical purgation. When the necessary cleansing has been accomplished, the patient's natural appetite and sense of wellbeing will return of their own accord. Then is the time to start a regimen of rebuilding.

Strong purgatives should not be used unless there's an acute or severe condition of excess that must be purged. Those who are relatively healthy and balanced will be made ill by the use of purgatives. Purgatives should also be matched in strength to the innate strength and vitality of the patient. Never use a stronger purgative or cleansing agent than is necessary to do the job.

An initial period of cleansing is not generally recommended for those in a very frail, emaciated or delicate state of health, however. These people need mild and gentle herbal tonics and dietary therapy to make them constitutionally stronger and resilient enough to undergo a cleansing regime.

Even where a regime of rebuilding, or recruitment, is clearly indicated, the physician, as the servant of Nature, cannot be too reckless or hasty. Acute cases of depletion should be replenished quickly. Someone suffering from acute dryness and dehydration, for example, should be fed with a rehydrating solution or herbal decoction immediately.

The same thing can also be said about cleansing or purgation. Slow, gentle cleansing while allowing the organism to detoxify gradually, in stages, is best for toxicity and plethora of long standing. Acute conditions of toxicity and congestion call for quick, decisive cleansing and purgation.

In cleansing or rebuilding, the physician simply mirrors or reverses, in a similar manner, the natural processes that led the patient into the disorder.

Therapeutic Modalities

In Persian Medicine, there are six major therapeutic modalities, or pathways to healing:

1) Dietary Therapy

2) Hygiene and Lifestyle Modification

3) Medicines, or Pharmacotherapy

4) Physiotherapy, or Bodywork

5) Hygienic Purification Therapies

6) Surgery, or Structural Modification of the Body

These six modalities of treatment are arranged in a natural priority. Dietary therapy is the gentlest, safest and least invasive; first, do everything you can to cure or ameliorate the condition through dietary means. Last on the list comes surgery, which is generally used as a last resort when all else fails.

These six modalities also fall into two distinct trinities, or triads, of therapy. The first three modalities are all administered by the patient himself in accordance with the physician's instructions. The last three are usually administered directly to the patient by the physician or therapist.

Of the first triad of therapies, to be administered by the patient himself under guidance from the physician, dietary modification comes first, supported by changes in lifestyle and hygiene habits. Only when these are insufficient should supplements and herbal medicines be resorted to. Of the second triad of therapies, to be administered by the physician or therapist, massage, physiotherapy and bodywork come first, and are often used as a preparatory measure for deeper forms of cleansing.

The dual therapies of massage with medicated oils, and sweating, are the basic modalities used to loosen and dislodge toxins from their deeply embedded, impacted state as a preparatory measure for flushing them out of the organism with the deeper hygienic purification therapies. This is what Persian Medicine is referring to when he declares:

"When one wishes to purge, he should put the body into a fluent state."

Detoxification through the hygienic purification therapies is one of the core therapeutic objectives of Persian Medicine, and can accomplish many healing miracles when appropriately done on those who have been properly prepared for it. The six hygienic purification methods are:

1) Sudation (sweating)

2) Diuresis (urination)

3) Emesis (vomiting)

4) Purgation (of the bowels)

5) Derivation (drawing out toxins through the skin)

6) Venesection (bloodletting)

And last on the list is surgery, to be done as a last resort only when all else fails. However, there are some conditions, usually involving trauma, injury or disfigurement, in which surgery is the essential first line of treatment.

Individualized Treatment

Avicenna once stated that Somtimes it's more important to know what kind of person has a disease than what kind of disease a person has. By this, he was referring primarily to considerations of the person's constitutional nature and temperament. The concept of the Four Temperaments forms the basis of all constitutional notions of diagnosis and treatment in Persian Medicine, which enables the physician to treat the patient, and not just the disease.

Because of individual differences of constitutional nature and temperament, no two people will manifest the signs and symptoms of a given disease in exactly the same way. Neither will they respond in exactly the same way to a given medicine or treatment regimen for that disease.

Each of the Four Temperaments responds differently to the various therapeutic modalities offered by Persian Medicine. But there are other factors to consider besides just the constitutional nature and temperament of the individual. Persian Medicine, as a holistic healing system, recognizes that no one exists in a vacuum; each individual lives in a dynamic interplay with his/her environment.

To Habit: This refers to the patient's particular habits of eating, living, activity, sleep and rest. The patient's daily habits in each of these areas have a profound influence on his state of health, and are often indicators of his constitutional nature and temperament. Accordingly, they must be duly considered by the physician in designing a treatment strategy that the patient is most likely to follow.

To Season: The various seasons of the year all have their characteristic influences on the patient's health and manifestation of disease signs and symptoms, due to their inherent nature and temperament. These seasonal influences have been discussed elsewhere in this website, in the Basic Principles and Hygiene sections.

To Country: Each kind of country, or natural environment, will have its characteristic temperament and influence, and will affect how the seasons manifest and express themselves throughout the course of the year. In a sunny subtropical or Mediterranean environment, or in a cold, dry, etc. The influence of the patient's natural environment will certainly affect the course of his/her therapy.

To Age: The various ages of the human lifespan can be likened to the various seasons of the year. This has been discussed in the Basic Principles section. In youth an individual is more sanguine in nature than he will ever be; in Middle Age, he is at his most melancholic. Such are the general rules and tendencies, of which, of course, there will be various and sundry individual variations.

Adjusting the Four Humors

Humoral imbalances are common. When a humor gets out of balance, the whole metabolism of the body is thrown off, and multiple signs and symptoms, many of which are seemingly unrelated, can appear in various parts of the body. And so, correcting underlying humoral imbalances can alleviate many health problems and complications.

Humoral imbalances can be of several different types, with each type indicating a certain basic therapeutic approach to restore balance:

The humor can be in excess or plethora, which can be either localized or systemic. In these cases, purgatives, or cleansing agents specific to the offending humor, are indicated.

The humor can be altered in temperament or corrupt in quality. This calls for medicines and treatments that purify and correct the qualitative corruption or morbidity of the humor.

The humor can be deficient, especially if it is one of the moist, flourishing humors - blood or phlegm / serous fluids. This calls for tonics and restoratives to nourish and replenish the humor back to its optimum level.

The humor can be poorly circulated and distributed throughout the body. In these cases, medicines or treatments that restore proper circulation and metabolism to the affected humor are called for.

Certain articles in this section discuss therapeutic approaches for correcting the various imbalances that can happen to each of the Four Humors.

Constitutional Strengthening and Support

One of the therapeutic approaches that Persian Medicine places a lot of faith in is restorative measures to strengthen and support the basic adaptive powers of the patient's physis, or constitution. In direct contrast to the allopathic approach of banishing or eradicating disease, this is the naturopathic approach of strengthening the vital forces of health and recuperation within the organism.

As the righteous forces of the patient's innate constitutional health and vitality are restored, many of his/her various complaints and infirmities will naturally ameliorate or disappear, just as the shadows of night flee before the rising sun. This therapeutic approach is health-specific rather than disease-specific. In modern holistic medicine, this therapeutic approach is called restorative or adaptogenic. It is based on a natural, wholesome diet in keeping with one's constitutional nature and temperament; health-promoting and stress-busting moderate exercise and fitness regimens coupled with beneficial lifestyle adjustments; and gentle yet effective herbal tonics and super foods.

Each one of the Four Temperaments, or basic constitutional types in Persian Medicine, has its own typical patterns of breakdown when challenged or under stress, both physical and psychological. These patterns of breakdown then indicate to the physician certain therapeutic approaches for shoring up and restoring constitutional strength and resiliency where it is needed the most.

These restorative constitutional treatments of Persian Medicine later became the basis for the Nature Cure treatments of health spas. The main objective is to let Mother Nature do the healing, and put back together a broken down constitution as only she knows how.

Therapeutic Goals and Priorities

In Persian Medicine, the usual therapeutic order of business is to work backwards, starting with resolving the most acute and short term manifestations of disease, and gradually correcting, as the means and opportunity present themselves, disease conditions of longer and more chronic standing and duration. The therapist tries to reverse the disease processes that led to the patient's infirm condition. No one would deny that acute flare-ups and crises demand the physician's immediate attention. If a fire is burning out of control, the physician must put it out. These acute crisis conditions include fever, acute infections, severe pain, vehement and uncontrolled diarrhea, colic, nausea and/or vomiting; seizures and convulsions; rashes and skin outbreaks; bleeding disorders, inflammatory crises and allergic or autoimmune reactions. These volatile acute conditions must be put under control before the patient's condition is stable enough to work steadily on the more chronic conditions.

These acute outbreaks need not always be from recently acquired conditions. Somtimes, morbid conditions held deeply and chronically within the organism can spawn acute flare-ups, or eruptions, when the conditions are right.

High on the physician's priority list must also be disease conditions that interfere with the Six Hygienic Factors, or the basic hygienic and lifestyle processes that empower healing and recovery. Conditions that generate acute, severe pain or discomfort, for example, can destruct sleep, which is essential for regeneration and healing.

Beyond these exigencies, therapeutic or healing goals and priorities are fairly flexible, and should be discussed between physician and patient. The patient's healing goals and priorities may not always be in his/her own best interests, however. It's up to the physician to diagnose and point out to his patient the existence of underlying serious or insidious pathologies that demand prompt and aggressive treatment.

Principles of dietary therapy

The Dietary Management of Disease

In Persian Medicine, dietary therapy and managing the patient's diet is an essential part of disease treatment, recovery and nursing the patient back to health. If we are to use the natural treatment methods and medicines of Persian Medicine, our success will be limited at best, and not thorough, lasting or complete unless we accompany our treatments with the right dietary measures. Indulging in the wrong food choices, at the wrong time, can spoil what otherwise would have been a faultless recovery.

Most conventional doctors practicing modern medicine are not very particular at all when it comes to diet, and don't give their patients much dietary advice, if any. The reasons for this are twofold:

1) Most people's dietary habits are so poor, irregular or unhealthy that the doctor feels that any dietary advice, if given, would simply be ignored. The busyness and demands of modern life often interfere with the proper, healthy regulation of diet as well.

2) The powerful pharmaceutical drugs given will usually produce the desired effect regardless of what the patient eats, by suppressing the symptoms and compel the patient's body into submission. There's a price to pay for this in overall health diminution over the long term, but most people don't care; they just want to pop a pill and forget it.

Diet and dietary therapy in Persian Medicine is divided into two basic parts:

1) The general rules and principles of healthy eating on a regular, daily basis, and the dietary management of one's temperament, or constitutional type.

2) Rules and principles regarding the dietary management of disease and the recovery process; this involves special, short-term diets and regimens designed to achieve certain specific therapeutic goals and objectives.

To put it another way, you could say that there are basically two kinds of diets:

1) A diet undertaken to maintain overall health and wellbeing on a regular basis over the long term.

2) A diet undertaken over the short term, or for a limited time period, designed to achieve certain specific therapeutic goals and objectives.

The first kind of diet was discussed in the article on Diet: Food and Drink in the Hygiene section. Here, we will deal with diets of the second kind, or those designed for disease management and health recovery.

Dietary Therapy in Acute Diseases

Dietary therapy is very important in the proper management of acute diseases. Particularly important is what Avicenna called the acute crisis, which is the acme, or climax, of an acute illness. At this stage of the acute disease process, the body is in a catharsis of elimination, so the worst thing to do is to burden it with digesting a lot of heavy foods.

When going through the acute crisis, Avicenna would feed his patients a liquid diet. This can consist of herbal teas or decoctions; broths made from green, root or sea vegetables; or fruit or vegetable juices diluted at least 50 / 50 with water. (Fruit and vegetable juices should not be mixed.) This will keep the patient well-hydrated with fluids while providing a basic amount of easily assailable vitamins, minerals, sugars and carbohydrates for basic energy and metabolic needs. If juices are used, they must be at room temperature or Hoter, not cold.

Persian Medicine explains his position on diet during the acute crisis in the following words:

"When the disease is at its height, it will then be necessary to use the slenderest diet."

A paroxysm is another word for an acute crisis episode. In other words, some acute diseases go through multiple, recurring or periodic crises. Whenever the patient is going through a crisis phase, we must administer only liquids, because the patient is eliminating toxins and pathogens from his system. If an acute disease has made its onset, but things are not yet at the crisis, or if the acute disease is in between paroxysms, or crisis phases, what do we do? What kind of diet do we administer to the patient? Avicenna explains: We must form a particular judgment of the patient, whether he will support the diet until the acme of the disease, and whether he will sink previously and not support the diet, or the disease will give way previously, and become less acute.

In other words, it's a judgment call. The physician must know the constitutional vigor and vitality of the patient and his/her energy reserves. On the other side of the equation, or battle, the physician must know the inherent seriousness and virulence of the acute disease the patient faces, and its probable course, or outcome.

Basically, you want to feed the patient a light diet throughout the course of the acute disease, but one sufficiently nutritious and hearty to support his/her energy levels sufficiently so that, when the crisis comes and we must retrench to a liquid diet, the patient has enough basic vitality and stamina to make it through. To support adequately, but not overburden the patient's digestive system is the guiding principle. The more severe and acute the symptoms, the slenderer and restricted must be the diet; conversely, the milder the symptoms, the more generous a diet we are allowed to give the patient. Avicenna explains:

When the disease is very acute, it is attended with extremely severe symptoms in its first stage; and therefore, an extremely attenuated diet must be used. When this is not the case, but it is allowable to give a more generous diet, we may depart as for from the severity of regimen as the disease, by its mildness, is removed from the extreme.

Correcting Humoral Imbalances with Diet

In Persian Medicine, as in other traditional healing systems, dietary therapy was seen to be an essential adjunct therapy to herbal medicine. The diet given to the patient had to help and assist, and not hinder, the natural herbal medicines he/she was taking. If the diet was not supporting the medicines and therapies administered to the patient, the success of the treatment would be partial or limited at best.

If the patient's body is eliminating excessive or superfluous humors, then a light diet of easily digestible foods is given. If the patient is suffering from nutritional or humoral deficiencies, or is recovering from an emaciating or debilitating illness, then a hearty, generous and full diet is given.

In recommending the right diet to a patient, the physician must always be mindful of the patient's pepsis, or digestion. Assessing the condition of the patient's pepsis, the physician never gives the patient food that he cannot digest and assimilate properly. Not only is the food important, but also so is the way it is prepared.

For example, a patient with a frail and delicate digestion may not be up to digesting and assimilating a slice of roast beef, but may be perfectly able to handle beef broth. Similarly, boiled potatoes are definitely easier to digest than fried potatoes.

If the patient's pepsis and digestion are weak, they may be strengthened and improved with the right foods, herbs and spices. Generally, these are pungent and aromatic. Improving the patient's pepsis and digestion is a basic, foundational therapeutic strategy in Persian Medicine because it is so important to the overall health and nutritional status of the patient.

Improving pepsis and digestion also helps to detoxify the organism and concoct, or consume and eliminate, morbid or superfluous humors. And a stronger, better pepsis helps to neutralize toxins and keep these morbid substances from accumulating.

Generally, foods with opposite qualities to the offending or unbalanced humor are given. Perhaps the best known examples are hot pungent foods like peppers, ginger or garlic to consume, concoct and eliminate excess phlegm. Then, the other half of this strategy for correcting humoral imbalances is to avoid foods that aggravate the offending humor. This way, you don't work against yourself and create any new humoral excesses or imbalances.

The particulars of dietary management of humoral imbalances will be discussed in subsequent articles in this section.

Dietary Therapy in Chronic Diseases

Generally speaking, chronic diseases require a diet that is hearty, wholesome and nutritious to build strength and vitality and strengthen weakened organs and systems. It is here that food can truly be our best medicine.

Above all, in chronic diseases, we must learn to allow sufficient generosity and flexibility in dietary food choices. Dietary restrictions where not absolutely necessary should be avoided, as a diet that is too strict will have a more limited spectrum or range of nutritional factors present in it.

The physician must be careful and vigilant in his assessment of the chronic disease sufferer, noting carefully which bodily organs and systems have become compromised and run down. Then he must carefully design therapeutic strategies, incorporating diet, for rebuilding these faculties and organ systems.

On the one hand, the physician must identify and eliminate problematic foods that are aggravating or contributing to the patient's chronic condition. An accurate assessment of the patient's constitutional nature and temperament is essential, because frequently the offending foods are those that are not suited to the patient's constitutional type.

When the patient's constitutional nature and temperament is of a dual type, a basic diet must be chosen that is suited to the primary temperament with nothing in it that will aggravate or unbalance the patient's secondary temperament. With three temperaments of roughly equal strength but one humor / temperament that are deficient, the weak one must be supplemented and strengthened with diet and tonic herbal therapy.

This whole idea of problematic foods ties in a lot with the modern medical concept of food allergies and intolerances. There is nothing wrong with using modern food allergy testing protocols; in many cases, these findings will help elucidate the subtler, more hidden aspects of the patient's constitutional nature and temperament.

The basic guidelines for the dietary management of each of the Four Temperaments have been given in the article on Diet in the Hygiene section. More about dietary therapy will be said in the articles on the therapeutic management of each of the Four Temperaments in this section.

And then there are those who have multiple food sensitivities and intolerances. In most of these cases, the patient's pepsis, or inherent vital forces of digestion and metabolism, needs to be strengthened and improved. Some food allergies and intolerances may prove to be deep-rooted and primary, but most of the secondary ones will ameliorate or disappear when pepsis is improved.

Then, once the problems involving food allergies and intolerances and problematic or aggravating foods have been resolved and handled, the physician can then select special therapeutic foods for the patient. The general rule is that any therapeutic food that rebuilds the compromised or weakened organ or system that does not aggravate the condition or humoral imbalance, or is in no other way problematic, may be used.

In all chronic conditions in which the digestive system and Natural Faculty have been weakened or compromised, rebuilding them is a top priority in rebuilding health. This is because the nutritional factors to rebuild every other organ or tissue in the body must first be digested and assimilated by the Natural Faculty. Chronic digestive disorders are those which are most immediately affected and improved by therapeutic changes in diet.

Herbal therapeutics and materia medica

The therapeutic use of herbs and herbal medicines in the world's great medical systems is guided by the principles and precepts of that system. In Persian Medicine, the therapeutic use of herbs is guided by the principles of humor, temperament and the Four Basic Qualities.

In herbal folk medicine, simple empirical experience guides the therapeutic use of herbs: this herb for this disease or symptom, that herb for that. But the world's great healing systems, including Persian Medicine, have developed sophisticated systems of herbal taste, temperature and energetics that guide the proper selection and use of herbs in the context of holistic healing.

Basic Principles of Herbal Therapeutics

1) The herbal medicines given should be opposite yet complementary in quality to the nature of the imbalance or disorder to bring the organism back into balance.

2) The herbal medicines given should be similar in the strength and degree of their influence to the severity of the imbalance or disorder to correct it to just the right degree.

3) The herbal medicines given should be pertinent to the humor, vital principle, and organ or body part being treated to properly target the disease or disorder.

4) The herbal medicines given for conditions of excess should cleanse, purge, or eliminate the morbid superfluities, whether gross or subtle, in a timely, precise, efficient manner.

5) The herbal medicines given for conditions of deficiency should nourish, supplement, strengthen or restore the affected or defective humor, organ, vital principle, and tissue or body part.

6) For conditions in between excess and deficiency caused by the faulty metabolism, circulation or distribution of a humor or vital principle, herbal medicines that balance, harmonize, circulate or metabolize the affected humor or vital principle, to the exact nature and degree that it is affected, should be given.

7) Herbal medicines to clear away any morbid excesses, impurities, obstructions or superfluities that remain should be given before the organism can be properly nourished, restored or rebuilt with the right herbal tonics and restoratives. In patients who are very weak, frail or emaciated, tonics and restoratives can be combined with gentle cleansers.

8) First, do no harm. The herbal medicines given should always be aimed at increasing the overall health, vitality, immunity of the organism as the s goal of treatment.

9) Learn as much as you can about an herb or herbal medicine before using it. Not only must you know its indications, or conditions for which it is used, but also its contraindications, or conditions that negate or prohibit its usage, as well as its potency, administration and dosage.

Herbal Qualities and Temperament

In Persian Medicine, everything or substance has its own inherent nature and temperament. This includes the herbs and other natural substances used as medicines.

The primary parameters used for measuring an herb or medicinal substance's nature, temperament and influence are the Four Basic Qualities. Of these Four Basic Qualities, the temperature polarity of Hot versus Cold is primary and most important, with Wet versus dry being of secondary importance. An herb or medicinal substance that is balanced or neutral in terms of these polarities, especially the primary polarity of temperature, is said to be temperate.

Herbs and medicinal substances whose qualities and temperament are opposite yet complementary to the nature of the disorder, to the same degree, are used to neutralize the disorder and bring the organism back into balance. Excessive heat must be cooled, cold must be Hoted or heated, and chills dispersed; dryness must be moistened, and dampness dried up.

The excessive or prolonged use of heating medicines will create a condition of secondary dryness. The excessive or prolonged use of cooling medicines will create a condition of secondary wetness.

In herbal treatments, preference must be given to herbs and medicines that are Hot or heating, because all living organisms generate heat, and cold is basically inimical to life. Cooling medicines should be used cautiously or sparingly, and only if definite signs of heat, fever, inflammation or hyper function are present, and only for as long as they are present.

Similarly, drying medicines should be used with more caution and prudence than moistening medicines, because moisture is necessary for life. However, this provision is not as stringent as the first or primary one; use each appropriately, according to the patient's signs and symptoms.

To help the physician or pharmacist measure more precisely the relative strength and potency of herbs and medicinal substances in formulating and administering herbs and herbal medicines, Persian Medicine assigned four degrees, or levels of potency, to each of the Four Basic Qualities, with the first degree being the mildest, and the fourth the most potent. The Persian Medicine Degree of the herb or medicine used must match the degree of severity of the disorder while being opposite yet complementary in quality.

Certain broad associations between the Four Basic Qualities and particular tastes and therapeutic properties of herbs and medicines can also be drawn. These are as follows:

Hot herbs and medicines stimulation and Hot the metabolism and disperse chills. Many are pungent and spicy in taste. Many are stimulants, expectorants, adaptogens and energy tonics.

Cold herbs and medicines sedate or slow down the metabolism and cool down fevers, heat and inflammation. Many are anti-inflammatory, antipyretics, refrigerants and sedatives. Many are also bitter in taste.

Wet herbs and medicines moisten, soothe and nourish. Many are demulcents, emollients and nutritive tonics. Many also have a bland or mildly sweet taste and an abundant supply of natural mucilage.

Dry herbs and medicines help the body eliminate excess fluids, phlegm and dampness. Many are expectorants, diuretics or astringents.

There are other qualities used to describe or characterize herbs and medicinal substances in Persian Medicine besides these basic four. Most of these qualities are also arranged in pairs of complementary opposites, and most have certain affinities to the basic four. Some of the most important of these qualities are: light / heavy; smooth / rough; sharp / dull; subtle / gross.

These basic qualities of herbs and medicines become the basis for their medicinal actions and effects. Medicinal substances have both qualities and actions inherent in them.

Herbal Actions

In herbal medicine, there are four basic levels of understanding the medicinal properties of an herb:

The most fundamental and primary level is understanding the herb's basic nature and temperament. This is what is often called taste, temperature and energetics.

The next level is that of herbal actions, or how herbs move, act and behave in the body after ingestion. This is the science of pharmacodynamics.

The third level is that of herbal effects, which is often expressed in the usual terms of diaphoretic, expectorant, stimulant, etc.

The fourth and final level is that of applications, or which conditions and disorders an herb treats or is used for. Knowledge concerning an herb's applications is usually passed down from centuries of clinical experience.

Let's look at some of the common therapeutic actions used to classify herbs in Persian Medicine:

Dispersing herbs and medicines have a floating, centrifugal energy that works from the interior outwards to release various toxins and pathogens through the skin and the surface of the body. Many of these herbs are pungent, acrid or aromatic. The medicinal effects of these herbs and medicines include: diaphoretic / sudorific, anodyne, discutient, resolvent.

Purging herbs and medicines vigorously eliminate accumulations of morbid humors or toxic matter from the body. Purging medicines are divided into two major groups: those which purge upwards, or emetics which provoke vomiting; and those which purge downwards, usually through the bowels, but also through the urinary tract.

Purgatives, especially the stronger ones, are very vigorous and extreme in their action, and should be used sparingly and cautiously, and only in cases of acute excess accumulation of morbid matter. If the excess or obstruction occurs above the navel, emetics are usually indicated; if below the navel, downwards purgatives are used. Being so vigorous in their action, purging medicines drain a lot of metabolic heat from the body; and so, their temperament is usually cold.

Softening herbs are also called emollients. Most are moistening and lubricating, neutral to mildly hot in temperament, mildly sweet or bland in taste, and rich in mucilage content. They embody the soft and smooth qualities, and are totally free of any roughness, harshness or astringency. Because of their nourishing mucilage content, many of these herbs are nutritive tonics.

Hardening herbs and medicines are cooling, drying and astringent, and are the opposite of softening medicines. They dry up excess moisture like a sponge, and thicken and congeal humors that are too thin, dispersed or attenuated. They also firm, tone up and consolidate not only organs and tissues that have become too loose and lax, but also vital principles and pneuma that have become too unfocused and dispersed as well.

Binding herbs and medicines are also cooling, drying and astringent, but their astringent action is stronger. Besides firming and toning up organs and tissues, binding astringents also stop or dry up excessive or abnormal secretions and excretions of the body, like bleeding, sweat, urine, diarrhea, leucorrhea and semen.

Glutinative medicines have a sticky, glutinous property that acts like glue to help regenerate tissue and aid in the healing of wounds and traumatic injuries. Many are classified as vulneraries or cicatrizants, and are used both topically in plasters, poultices, liniments and wound dressings as well as internally as first aid for injuries and trauma.

Loosening medicines relax and release nervous and muscular tensions. They are temperate to hot or heating in temperament. Their loosening action has a lot in common with dispersing medicines, except that they work not on the surface, but on the deeper organs and tissues of the body. Like the dispersing medicines, most loosening medicines also have strong aromatic principles. Loosening medicines that release nervous and muscular tensions are called nervines, sedatives or antispasmodics. Loosening medicines that ease the flow of vital energy in the lungs and chest and stop spasmodic coughs are pectorals and antitussives. Loosening medicines that release colic, distension, and smooth muscle tension in the gut are called carminatives and stomachic.

Attenuating medicines cut through and thin out excessively thick or congealed humors. Most of them have a Hot or heating temperament and a pungent or acrid taste. Attenuating medicines are also called scraping medicines, because many scrape away accumulations of metabolic excess residues in the body, like high blood sugar and high cholesterol. Other attenuating medicines simply thin and liquefy excessively thick and congealed humors like phlegm or blood to aid in their circulation, metabolism or expulsion.

Concocting herbs and medicines are those that promote the ripening, metabolism, flow and secretion of various humors and vital fluids of the body, improving their physiological function within the organism, as well as facilitating the expulsion of their morbid superfluities.

Herbs that concoct or regenerate the blood are usually pungent and aromatic.

Herbs that concoct phlegm are called expectorants, and are basically of two kinds: heating pungent herbs that resolve and eliminate cold phlegm, and cooling herbs and medicines that dissolve tough, thick, hot, dry phlegm.

Herbs that concoct, circulate or remove obstructions to the flow of lymph and serous fluids are called lymphatic; many are also mild diuretics that improve body fluid metabolism and aid the body in excreting superfluities thereof.

Herbs that concoct and improve the flow and secretion of bile, or the Choleric humor, by the liver and gall bladder are called choleretics and cholagogues. Most are cooling and bitter, and are also called bitters or bitter tonics.

Since black bile, or the Melancholic humor, is a recognized clinical entity in Persian Medicine, there are also special herbs that concoct and dispel morbid excesses of black bile from the body.

Digestive herbs and medicines use this concocting action to concoct and digest accumulations of stagnant, undigested food in the digestive tract. They clear the stomach and move the bowels. Being pungent, acrid or sour, many digestive herbs are rich in digestive enzymes.

Herbs that resist poison are strongly heating, and vigorously stimulation the metabolism to neutralize and eliminate poisons and toxins.

Many say that herbal medicine first grew and evolved as an effort to find effective antidotes to the bites of venomous snakes and insects, as well as other poisons. Often, these antidotes were combined into complex electuary or medicinal paste formulations called Mithridates.

Stimulant herbs are those that are strongly heating, which vigorously stimulation the digestive and metabolic fires of the body. Their applications are threefold:

1) To concoct and eliminate morbid superfluities of cold, wet phlegm due to their heating and drying action;

2) To stimulation the stomach and digestion, and to neutralize and eliminate cold, heavy, thick toxic residues of rich foods and meats;

3) To hot the interior and disperse chills in colds and respiratory infections.

In contrast to these herbal stimulants, many commonly available stimulants, like Coffee, Tea and Cola drinks, although herbally derived, are rich in caffeine. They stimulation not the whole metabolism, but just the nervous system, and their abuse can lead to empty, ungrounded energy and nervous burnout.

Drawing medicines draw out pus and toxins, releasing them through the surface of the body. Many of these substances are used topically in plasters, poultices and cataplasms. They usually draw out these pathogens due to their Hot, heating action or their astringency. Drawing medicines that are extremely heating and draw out hot, purulent toxins through the skin by sympathy are called vesicants or counterirritants. Through topical application, they form blisters and abscesses, or pustules, whose toxic matter is then drained through lancing.

You may have noticed that there is a considerable degree of overlap in these herbal action categories. Indeed, a single herb may exhibit multiple actions, as a broad, diverse spectrum of medicinal actions and effects is typical of the herbal kingdom. Like people, herbs, as creatures of Nature, each have their own unique and complex constitutional makeups of qualities, actions and effects.

Eliminative Herbal Therapies

Persian Medicine stated that diseases of fullness, or repletion, are cured by depletion, which is elimination. Eliminative herbal therapies are indicated in all disorders of excess, superfluity and obstruction.

There are many different kinds of morbid humors and other forms of toxic matter, which can be either systemic or localized in virtually any organ or part of the body. The eliminative herbal therapies used must be specific both to the kind of toxic superfluous matter being eliminated as well as to its location, eliminating these superfluities or obstructions through the most appropriate organ, channel or orifice. Besides morbid humors and other toxic matter, eliminative herbal therapy also includes eliminating chills, drafts, or other forms of dystemper.

The eliminative therapy used must also be similar in the degree of its strength to the degree of acuteness or severity of the excess or obstruction. In addition, consideration must also be given to the patient's constitutional strength and resiliency, and to how vigorous of a purging he/she is able to withstand. All eliminative herbal therapies, by provoking a catharsis, drain some amount of metabolic heat and energy from the organism in doing so; the stronger the purging or catharsis, the more metabolic heat and energy are drained.

And so, the wise herbal therapist prefers to conserve the basic metabolic heat and energy of the patient as much as possible by giving preference to the gentler forms of eliminative therapy, and using the more vigorous, drastic or extreme forms only when absolutely necessary. The general rule is to never use an eliminative therapy or treatment that is stronger than what's absolutely necessary to do the job. A gentler, more gradual cleansing is usually easier on the basic metabolism and homeostasis of the organism than a quick, extreme catharsis. However, there may be acute crisis situations when vigorous, decisive measures are called for. To cleanse the body of morbid matter, eliminative herbs must work through the various eliminative organs of the body. These are mainly as follows:

1) The skin and its pores;

2) The lungs and respiratory tract;

3) The stomach, digestive tract and bowels;

4) The liver, gall bladder and hepatobiliary tract;

5) The kidneys, bladder and genitourinary tract.

Most of the eliminative herbs can be used to facilitate, support or enhance one or more of the Six Hygienic Purification Therapies of Persian Medicine:

1) Diaphoresis - Sweating

2) Emesis - Vomiting

3) Diuresis - Urination

4) Purgation - Evacuation through the bowels and GI tract

5) Venesection - Bloodletting

6) Derivation - Drawing out toxins through the skin

Morbid humors or other superfluous toxic matter must be removed through one or more of the eliminative organs. Dystempers and imbalances of qualities and energies can be neutralized by herbs with opposite yet complementary qualities and energies.

In our discussion of eliminative therapies, we will be starting with herbs that work on a more superficial or subtle level first, and progressing to herbs that are deeper and more substantial in their therapeutic actions.

Diaphoretics are herbs that disperse exogenous pathogenic factors such as wind, cold and heat from the surface and superficial regions of the body through sweating. Most of them are rich in fragrant, volatile essential oils that are cleansing and disinfecting, and are released through the pores of the skin. Diaphoretics are generally either Hot and Stimulating or cooling and sedating; a few are rather neutral or temperate, containing aspects of both.

Hot, Stimulating Diaphoretics are generally used to treat colds caused by catching a chilly draft, with symptoms of coughs and lung congestion, nasal blockage, no sweating or furtive sweating, chills, or chills and fever, muscular aches and pains, and an aversion to wind and cold. Cooling, Sedating Diaphoretics are generally used to treat colds of a hot, febrile nature, caused by catching a hot draft or evil wind, with symptoms of fever, profuse sweating, headache, irritability, sore throat, red eyes and swollen glands.

To induce sweating, diaphoretic teas must be drunk hot. Because sweating opens the pores and drains more metabolic energy from the body than you realize, it's a good idea to keep yourself bundled up in Hot, protective clothing, and to have a light soup or barley gruel, about 20 minutes to a half hour after sweating.

Other superficial dispersing therapies that are very closely allied to diaphoretic sweating therapy are Discutient and Anodyne therapy. Many diaphoretic herbs can also be used as discutients and others as anodynes, and there is a high degree of overlap between them.

Discutients are herbs that discuss, or promote the eruption and release of measles or other skin rashes through sweating. Most are also cooling, sedating diaphoretics, or neutral, temperate ones. Peppermint and other diaphoretic teas can be drunk from time to time to cleanse the pores and keep the skin beautiful and healthy.

Anodynes are hot diaphoretics that are more hot and not so strongly diaphoretic, which Hot the muscular peripheral layer of the body, improve circulation and metabolic heat, and disperse cold, damp rheumatic vapors with their hot aromatic principles, relieving muscular tension and rheumatic aches and pains. Besides drinking them as hot herb teas, their essential oils can also be put into medicated massage oils.

Herbs that clear heat are those that subdue fevers and inflammation and dispel hot, Choleric vapors from the body. Herbs that subdue fevers are called febrifuges, whereas those that dispel inflammation are called anti-inflammatories. Most of these herbs are cold or cooling in temperament, although a few are neutral, temperate or slightly hot.

Febrifuges are of many kinds, and used to subdue different types of fevers. This group includes herbs that contain salicylates, which, in addition relieving ardent and ephemeral fevers are also anti-inflammatories.

Antiperiodic are herbs that dispel intermittent or periodic fevers like the tertian or quatrain fevers caused by morbid accumulations of yellow and black bile. Not surprisingly, many of these herbs are also bitter tonics and cholagogues.

Some fevers are subdued directly, but many fevers are broken with a sweat. And so, many diaphoretics are also febrifuges, especially the ones that are more neutral to cooling in temperament. But if there is a fever with chills, Stimulating, Hot diaphoretics are indicated. Many febrifugal herbs have some diaphoretic effect, and to emphasize this aspect, the herbs are given as hot teas.

Anti-inflammatories cover a broad spectrum of herbs, and like herbs with beneficial effects on the liver, there are also many fine herbs with some beneficial effect on subduing inflammation. As with febrifuges, most of these herbs are cold or cooling in temperament, although some are temperate or hot.

So, vast and multifaceted are the range and diversity of anti-inflammatory effects obtained by herbs that pharmaceutical anti-inflammatory drugs seem crude and primitive by comparison. Modern medicine is truly worse off in this respect for its anti-herbal bias. There are herbs for stronger or weaker, acute or chronic states of inflammation, as well as those that work systemically versus those that relieve inflammation in specific organs, tissues or body parts.

Some anti-inflammatory herbs may not be strongly or directly anti-inflammatory, but nevertheless help to improve the organism's resistance to inflammation. These herbs are called inflammomodulatory, and many herbs have this capability, to a greater or lesser extent.

Anti-inflammatory herbs are mostly cooling and drying in temperament, with the coldness subduing the heat, redness and pain of inflammation, and the dryness dispersing the swelling and congestion. Many anti-inflammatory herbs are quite bitter in taste, although quite a few others have a marked astringency to them. Both the bitter and astringent tastes are cooling and drying in temperament.

Stimulants are the complementary opposites of the febrifuges and anti-inflammatories in that they have a strongly heating temperament. Stimulants hot the interior and stoke the digestive and metabolic fires of the body to disperse chills, as well as dispel cold, moist Phlegmatic humors and vapors, or the damp, turbid toxic residues of a cold, weak pepsis and digestion. These herbs have already been discussed, and examples given, in the section on Herbal Actions.

Expectorants are closely allied to stimulants in that they dissolve and expel phlegm; to do this, most, but not all, have a hot or heating temperament. Actually, expectorants can be broadly subdivided into hot or heating expectorants that expel cold phlegm, and cooling, moistening expectorants that dissolve and liquefy hot, dry phlegm, facilitating its expectoration. And again, some expectorants can contain aspects of both.

There's a third class of expectorants that aid expectoration and relieve phlegm congestion in the lungs and chest by facilitating the flow of vital energy and fluids in that part of the body.

Next, we turn our attention to the bowels, which is what purgatives are all about. A laxative is a mild purgative, which facilitates bowel movements, whereas a true purgative is stronger. Somtimes, the difference between the two therapeutic actions is merely a matter of dosage; smaller doses tend to be milder and more like laxatives, whereas larger doses tend to be stronger and more purgative.

In cleansing and moving the bowels, our aim is to relieve and correct constipation, or the excessive retention of wastes in the colon and intestines, which has been called the Mother of All Diseases. In laxative and purgative therapy, there are three golden rules that must be followed:

1) Try to relieve constipation with dietary measures first.

2) Address and correct the root cause of the constipation.

3) Always use the gentlest herb, formula or medicine that will do the job to avoid dependency.

We will begin our discussion of herbs and medicines to purge and move the bowels with the gentler agents first, and then progress to the more vigorous and drastic ones.

Aperients have a mild loosening or relaxing effect on the bowels, and gently nudge them to have smooth and natural bowel movements. Some aperients gently stimulation the flow of bile, which is the body's own natural laxative.

Bulk Laxatives are those that gently provoke the defecation reflex through their content of soluble fiber, which expands to provide bulk in the intestines in the presence of water.

Lubricant Laxatives are those that gently lubricate the bowels to move through their softening demulcent or emollient effects. They are very useful in constipation due to dryness or withering of the bowels, with hard, dry stools; many of them are also stool softeners. Others are actually lubricating oils or oil rich seeds.

Stimulant Laxatives provoke a vigorous defecation reflex by Stimulating or mildly irritating the bowels. Because of their vigorous purging action, most stimulant laxatives are cold in temperament, and drain considerable metabolic energy from the body and the digestive tract. Many abuse harsh stimulant laxatives, developing a dependency on them when they should have used dietary measures or the milder laxatives or aperients instead.

The exact effect that these stimulant laxatives have also depends on their formulation, preparation, administration and dosage. In smaller doses, and combined with other herbs, the first three stimulant laxatives on the list can also function as cholagogues that promote the flow of bile, for example. The medium of administration is also important; tinctures, or alcoholic extracts, lessen the downwards purging nature of stimulant laxatives.

Correctives are herbs or medicines that soften, moderate or correct the harsh action of stimulant laxatives and other strong purgatives, relieving the intestinal discomfort, spasm, colic and griping that they can cause. Correctives are usually softening demulcents or emollients, loosening carminatives or Stimulating digestive tonics.

Cathartics are drastic purging agents that cause rapid and vigorous evacuations from the stomach and bowels, and also from the urinary tract as well. Some cause purging both upwards, as in vomiting, as well as downwards through the bowels and urinary tract.

Emetics are herbs that purge upwards from the stomach, causing vomiting. Emesis is one of the Six Hygienic Purification Therapies of Persian Medicine, and can be very beneficial for chronic phlegm congestion in the stomach, lungs and respiratory tract.

Vermifuges are herbs that purge the intestines of worms and parasites. They are best used under medical supervision, including an initial diagnosis through stool sample, as well as monitoring and follow-up testing. Vermifuges vary from gentle to potent or harsh in the inherent strength of their action. They are also used in combination with the right adjuvants and correctives, not only to soften and moderate their own action if they are harsh or drastic, but also to loosen and lubricate the bowels to facilitate the expulsion of the worms and parasites.

According to Persian Medicine, those whose bodies are heavily encumbered by great accumulations of morbid humors and other forms of toxic matter are usually those who have the greatest problems with worms and other forms of parasite infestation. Not only do these accumulations of morbid humors and toxic matter inhibit the natural immunity of the organism, but they also provide the food for the parasites to feed on. If there are intestinal parasites, a systemic deep cleansing of the entire organism is usually indicated.

Adjusting and regulating blood

In Persian Medicine, blood, or the Sanguine humor, is the essence of life and health. To maintain vibrant youth and good health, it's important to cleanse this most vital of all humors, and keep it in balance through constant regeneration and renewal.

Herbs are the main therapeutic agents used to adjust and regulate blood, or the Sanguine humor. Also venesection or bloodletting is used to adjust the Sanguine humor by draining off the excess, and to alter the dynamics of its flow. Cupping, or Hejamat, either wet or dry, is another important therapy for dispersing or redirecting the flow of blood. The therapeutic principle here is derivation, or drawing blood away from a point of congestion or stagnation.

In herbal medicine, herbs that adjust, cleanse or purify the blood are broadly referred to as alterative, because they bring about profound alterations in a person's state of health for the better. Alteratives are of many different kinds, and bring about many different kinds of beneficial changes in the blood, according to their indications.

Diet: Eating to Build Healthy Blood

Blood is the very essence of Life and Health, and is perfect nourishment perfectly digested. As the first humor to arise, blood is also the first humor to be replenished and regenerated from the food we eat. Eating a balanced, wholesome, nourishing diet is the best way to generate healthy and vital blood for optimum health.

Eating meat generates a great abundance of blood, but the down side is that it will be too thick, acidic and filled with toxic residues. Eating meat is only necessary two to three times per week at the most to keep the blood robust and healthy.

Those of a Sanguine temperament, who naturally generate an abundance of blood, have an easy time being vegetarians.

Those of a Choleric temperament, whose blood tends to get too hot, Choleric and acidic, need an abundance of fresh fruits and vegetables to cleanse their blood; since their digestion is generally strong and robust, Choleric usually have an easy time being vegetarians.

Those of a Phlegmatic temperament can go either way, meat eater or vegetarian; a little meat can be good to stimulation their metabolic heat and digestive fire. Those of a Melancholic temperament tend to have the hardest time being pure vegetarians, since their weak, colicky, delicate digestions make them most prone to malnutrition and anemia.

Other Therapies for Adjusting and Regulating the Blood

Besides herbs and diet, there are other important therapies that Persian Medicine uses to adjust and regulate blood, or the Sanguine humor.

To remove excesses and localized congestions of the blood, Persian Medicine uses venesection, or bloodletting. Besides directly puncturing a vein and draining the excess blood into a bowl, two other forms of bloodletting are done: leeching, and wet cupping, or scarification and cupping. A more thorough discussion of venesection or bloodletting can be found on the Hygienic Purification Therapies page in the Therapies section.

Hejamat, or Cupping is the application of suction cups to specific points on the body to relieve localized congestions of blood in those areas. Cupping can be done either wet, which is scarification and cupping, a form of bloodletting; or dry cupping, which is the simple application of suction cups to draw out and disperse deep seated congestions of blood. Again, please refer to the appropriate page in the Therapies section. Derivation is the drawing out of morbid pus and toxic matter from the blood by the localized application of vesicant and counterirritant plasters to the affected area.

Adjusting and regulating phlegm and serous fluids

The Phlegmatic humor is divided into two portions: phlegm and serous fluids. Phlegm is accumulated mucus, the secretions of the body's mucous membranes. The serous fluids are the deeper clear fluids of the body - plasma, lymph, interstitial fluids, synovial fluid and cerebrospinal, pericardial and pleural fluids. All these fluids and mucous secretions are manifestations of the

Water element in the human body, and readily respond to and influence each other. If one of them is aggravated or out of balance, it will affect the others as well.

What unites all the various Phlegmatic fluids of the body is their common temperament: Cold and Wet. So, the general rule is that heating and/or drying substances tend to reduce the Phlegmatic humor, whereas cooling and/or moistening substances tend to increase it.

However, there are also many other factors that can complicate the clinical picture. Once phlegm is generated and accumulates in excess, it can easily stagnate and be unduly retained in the body, due to its passive, sluggish nature. And during the course of its retention, it can be influenced by all kinds of pathogenic factors that can alter its qualities and consistency, requiring other therapeutic qualities and approaches to remove it. Lymph and serous fluids, especially when chronically excessive or aggravated, can be complicated by other pathogenic factors as well. The organs that regulate their metabolism and excretion, such as the spleen, lungs or kidneys, can also become weak or devitalized.

Working with Phlegm

The first line of treatment in any phlegm reducing regimen must be dietary. Foods that generate excess phlegm, and foods and drink that cool or weaken the Digestive Fire and Metabolic Heat of the Natural Faculty, must be avoided. These include cooling, moistening foods like cucumbers and melons; cold drinks and juices; milk and dairy products; sugar and sweets; and refined white sugars and starches.

Herbs that stimulation the Digestive Fire and Metabolic Heat of the Natural Faculty with their heating, drying qualities are called stimulants. By having a heating, drying, and Stimulating effect on humor generation in the liver, stimulants adjust the metabolism so that less phlegm is generated. By their antipathy of temperament to phlegm, these heating stimulants burn off and evaporate excess moisture and phlegm from the body.

Rather than focusing on one part of the body, the action of most stimulants is systemic, to concoct, dissolve and eliminate excess phlegm throughout the organism by Stimulating circulation, digestion and metabolism. Galen was a great believer in the power of heating stimulants to concoct and dispel excess phlegm, and included many of them in his herbal formulas.

Expectorants are herbs that help the body eliminate excess phlegm, usually by expectorating or coughing it up from the lungs and respiratory tract. Due to the cold, wet nature of phlegm, most of these herbs are hot and drying in temperament. However, expectorants that facilitate the expulsion of excess phlegm by liquefying or attenuating phlegm that has become thickened or toughened by pathogenic heat and/or dryness can be moistening, and either temperate or slightly cooling in temperature.

Expectorant herbs that are strongly heating tend to specialize in removing watery, insipid phlegm, which is the coldest in temperament of all the types of phlegm.

Thick, slimy white or clear phlegm usually originates from a cold, weak, atonic stomach and digestion, and then gets transferred or spreads to the lungs via the gastro pulmonary reflex. The expectorants in this category are moderately Hot and drying in temperament, and have a dual action - not only facilitating the expectoration of excess phlegm from the lungs and respiratory tract, but also improving digestion by concocting and dissolving excess phlegm from the stomach and GI tract.

Somtimes, aggravations of coldness and phlegm clog the delicate respiratory passages, obstructing the free flow of pectoral pneuma or vital energy, provoking breathing difficulties or spasmodic coughing. For these conditions, expectorants with a loosening action that opens the airways, deepens breathing, and reduces spasmodic coughing are called for.

Liquefying expectorants are used to facilitate the expectoration of tough, thickened phlegm that has been so altered by pathogenic heat and dryness.

Although excess and congestion is the more common problem in dealing with phlegm, one can also suffer from a deficiency of these mucous secretions as well. In the respiratory tract, this would produce conditions like hoarseness, sore throat and a dry, hacking cough.

Emesis for Excess Phlegm

One of the most powerful ways to eliminate excess phlegm from the body is by emesis, or therapeutic vomiting. Emesis eliminates excess phlegm from the stomach, lungs, chest, respiratory tract and head by powerfully activating the gastro pulmonary reflex, to purge upwards. Emesis has been found to be effective in cases of chronic bronchitis, lung congestion and asthma. Many of the herbs used to provoke emesis are very heating and drying, and therefore fit the general profile of an anti-phlegm herb. Emetic herbs are quite potent, and are best used under medical supervision.

There are two other reasons why emesis is best performed under medical supervision: First of all, the trained clinical eye of a physician is best fit to discern who would be a good candidate for emesis, and who wouldn't. Secondly, those who suffer from psychosomatic eating disorders like bulimia are prone to abuse emesis.

Working with Serous Fluids

With phlegm, the most common problems that the physician must deal with are generally those of excess. With serous fluids, which form the bulk of the moist, flourishing Phlegmatic humor, deficiency is just as much of a common problem as excess.

Deficiency conditions of the serous fluids are essentially various forms of dehydration, either acute or chronic. Excess conditions of the serous fluids are essentially various forms of water retention, edema, and lymphatic congestion and obstruction. In addition to these deficiency and excess conditions, you can also have various toxic conditions of the lymph and serous fluids, in which the Waters of Life have become polluted.

Here again, to keep the serous fluids, or the deeper Waters of Life healthy, the first line of treatment should be dietary. Over two-thirds of our body consists of Water, or various types of fluids, so keeping them balanced, pure and healthy is a top health priority. And the foods that work most directly on preserving the health, balance and integrity of the serous fluids and other bodily fluids are fruits and vegetables, preferably fresh or minimally cooked and processed.

Fresh fruits and vegetables also alkalize the blood and serous fluids, which need to be slightly alkaline to be balanced in PH. But because so many people consume so few fresh fruits and

Vegetables, many people suffer from acidosis, or a chronically acidic condition of the blood and serous fluids.

Fresh vegetables alkalize the blood and serous fluids directly, since they themselves are alkaline. Most fresh fruits, especially the tart or sour ones, are themselves acidic, but alkalize the blood and serous fluids indirectly through their diuretic effect, which increases the elimination of acidic toxins.

Here again, the general rule for working with the serous fluids, whether with foods or with herbs, is that cooling and/or moistening foods and herbs tend to increase or nourish the serous fluids, whereas heating and/or drying foods and herbs tend to reduce serous fluids, or keep them balanced and in check by improving their circulation and metabolism.

Nourishing the Serous Fluids

Foods that have a nourishing, increasing effect on the serous fluids are mainly cooling and moistening fruits and vegetables.

Herbs that nourish or increase the serous fluids in conditions of deficiency or dehydration are called serous tonics, and generally have a moderately cooling and/or moistening temperament. Since many of these herbs can also soothe and moisten the mucous membranes, there's a high degree of overlap between them and the demulcents and emollients.

Nutritive tonics, or serous tonics, occupy an esteemed and valuable place in herbal medicine, especially in facilitating recovery from the ravages of serious or prolonged febrile or wasting diseases. Fenugreek seeds, although basically hot and drying in temperament, also have nutritive mucilaginous constituents in them; Avicenna used Fenugreek seed to facilitate convalescence from serious or prolonged respiratory tract infections.

Reducing Serous Fluids

When it comes to reducing or eliminating excess serous fluids from the body, the main vehicle for their release is through the urine; and so, most herbs that reduce or eliminate excess serous fluids have a diuretic effect. Secondarily, sweating through diaphoretics can also eliminate excess serous fluids.

All diuretics are drying in temperament and action, since they reduce the overall fluid level in the body through diuresis. Cooling diuretics, in addition to eliminating fluids, also cool and detoxify, eliminating excess heat and choler from the blood and serous fluids. Hot diuretics, as well as those that are moderate or temperate in temperature, generally eliminate excess fluids by improving their circulation and metabolism; it's these Hot and drying diuretics that are most directly remedial for excesses of serous fluids and the Phlegmatic humor.

Venous blood, like the Phlegmatic humor, is also Cold and Wet, or cool and moist, in temperament. In addition, since the lymphatic system drains back into the venous system, poor venous circulation and return often accompanies water retention, edema and lymphatic obstruction. So, many diuretics that improve the circulation and metabolism of serous fluids also work to improve venous circulation and return.

The main organs that regulate the circulation, metabolism and excretion of water and serous fluids are the lungs, liver, spleen and kidneys. Each of these organs has certain characteristic fluid retention signs and symptoms associated with it.

The lungs, which are closely associated with the heart, are associated with swelling and fluid retention in the chest, lungs, arms, hands, face and upper body. When associated with severe conditions of congestive heart failure, this is called cardiac edema.

The liver is often associated with swelling and bloating in the abdominal region which is worse after eating. This kind of edema is also associated with portal hypertension, or poor venous return to the liver from the intestines through the veins of the hepatic portal system.

The spleen purifies and metabolizes the lymph, which is one of the most important serous fluids. Splenic edema is associated with lymphatic toxicity, congestion and obstruction, and generally pervades the whole body, right below the skin. Congestion and poor metabolism of the spleen and lymph is also associated with chronic damp, oozing skin conditions like weeping eczema.

If the kidneys are weak and devitalized, the water retention will be mainly below the waist, especially in the knees, ankles and feet. Chronic edema in the low back, hips and loins is also associated with rheumatic and arthritic conditions, and so many of these herbs are also antirheumatic in their effects.

Some diuretics eliminate excesses of phlegm and serous fluids through their strong Hot, Stimulating effect on digestion and metabolism.

When it comes to using diuretics, it's generally best to stick to the milder and gentler ones, especially until you get more proficiency in herbal medicine.

Adjusting and regulating the choleric humor

The Choleric humor, also known as the Bilious humor, is hot and dry in temperament. Since its primary quality is Hot, the vast majority of herbs and medicines used to adjust and regulate the

Choleric humor when it is aggravated or out of balance are Cold or cooling in nature.

When the Choleric humor is out of balance or aggravated, the most commonly seen clinical manifestations are irritation, inflammation, swelling, jaundice, bilious disorders, acid indigestion, fevers, and purulent, bleeding and ulcerous conditions.

Therefore, herbs and medicines used to treat aggravations of the Choleric humor commonly have the following therapeutic properties: demulcent, anti-inflammatory, antiphlogistic, antihistamine, choleretic, cholagogue, hepatic, aperitive or bitter tonic, antacid, febrifugal, antipyretic, resolvent, detoxifying, hemostatic, styptic and astringent.

Acute manifestations of Choleric aggravation and imbalance, like fever, swelling, inflammatory crises or bleeding ulcers, can be quite serious and urgent, and demand immediate therapeutic intervention.

Even the smoldering embers of a chronic or recalcitrant Choleric condition like chronic gastroenteritis, inflamed and bleeding gums, or various other chronic inflammatory or bilious conditions can rob your body of the harmony and integration it needs to heal, and insidiously eat away at the organism's reserves of vitality and immunity. They can also disrupt the wholeness and integrity of the body's overall humoral balance and fluid metabolism. Correcting these chronic Choleric imbalances and disorders is therefore equally important.

Basic Principles for Adjusting and Correcting Yellow Bile

Yellow Bile can become morbid or corrupted in the following ways:

- It can be softened by admixture with watery phlegm and dampness;
- It can be corrupted by admixture with thick, toughened phlegm;

• It can be thickened and dried by chronic or excessive heat, or by admixture with
• Morbid Black Bile;
• It can be charred black, or oxidized due to excessive Metabolic Heat.

These morbid varieties of Yellow Bile are arranged in order, starting with the coldest and wet in temperament, progressing to the hottest and dry. Accordingly, the herbs and therapies used to resolve and eliminate the colder, moister varieties of morbid Yellow Bile must be hotter and dryer in temperament, whereas the herbs and therapies used to resolve and eliminate the hotter, dryer varieties must be colder and moister in temperament.

In addition, each one of these morbid forms of Yellow Bile, especially the thinner, softer varieties, can assume a subtle, vaporous form and be carried through the bloodstream to affect virtually any part of the body. If the morbid Yellow Bile remains in its gross form, it tends to remain close to its site of origin in the liver and hepatobiliary tract, as well as the middle and lower GI tract.

The herbs and therapies used to treat morbid Yellow Bile in its subtle vaporous form focus more on the non-digestive manifestations of Choleric imbalance, such as fever, irritation, inflammation, ulceration, swelling, purulent conditions and bleeding disorders. Accordingly, these herbs and therapies are predominantly febrifugal, antipyretic, antiperiodic, anti-inflammatory, astringent, styptic, antiphlogistic, antipurulent and hemostatic.

The herbs and therapies used to treat the hepatic, bilious and digestive manifestations of Choleric imbalance are most commonly choleretic, cholagogue, hepatic, aperitive or bitter tonic, antiulcerative, anticatarrhal, aperient and laxative.

What the vast majority of the herbs used to treat Choleric or bilious disorders, as well as the various systemic manifestations of excessive heat and choler have in common is the bitter taste.

This is true especially of herbs that treat the various digestive and hepatobiliary manifestations of Choleric imbalance.

The bitter taste is very hot in nature; it is also very soothing and detoxifying. In addition to Stimulating and promoting the flow of bile, the bitter taste, as exemplified in the bitter tonics of herbal medicine, has an almost magical ability to regenerate and restore proper pepsis when it has become deranged or dysfunctional due to imbalances and aggravations of the Choleric humor.

After the bitter taste, the astringent taste can also be very therapeutic and beneficial for correcting certain imbalances and disorders of the Choleric humor. The astringent taste is cooling, which is a necessary prerequisite for correcting Choleric imbalances and aggravations, but it is also drying, making it useful for bringing down swelling caused by histamine reactions secondary to inflammation. The binding action of astringents is also very useful for closing wounds and ulcerations, and in stopping bleeding due to excessive heat and choler in the blood.

The pungent taste, also known as spicy, is a valuable adjunct or auxiliary to the bitter taste when it comes to concocting and resolving the colder, moister forms of morbid Yellow Bile, which are due to admixtures with various types of phlegm. With bitter and pungent herbs, the bitter taste cools down and resolves the aggravated heat and choler, while the pungent taste concocts, resolves and eliminates the phlegm by Stimulating pepsis. Since bilious agues, or intermittent fevers are caused by a morbid softening of the Choleric humor due to admixture with damp, thin, watery forms of phlegm, many bitter and pungent herbs are also antiperiodic that resolve these types of fevers.

With the hotter, dryer varieties of morbid Yellow Bile, or with morbid Yellow Bile that has become admixed with thickened , toughened forms of phlegm, bitter herbs with a secondary moistening, emollient, attenuating, liquefying quality are used. Once this liquefaction or attenuation has been accomplished, these morbid excesses of Yellow Bile can be easily expelled by the eliminative organs of the body, chiefly the kidneys, liver and hepatobiliary system.

Throughout the remainder of this article, I will be introducing you to various herbs and therapies for correcting Choleric imbalances that fit the general profiles outlined here. According to the principles of Persian Medicine, Yellow Bile takes at least three days to ripen. So, in treating Choleric and bilious disorders, the course of treatment should take at least three days, with at least five days or more for difficult or recalcitrant cases.

Dietary Therapy for Choleric Disorders

For Choleric disorders, as for those of any other humor, the first line of treatment and prevention is dietary. For those of a Choleric temperament, who are prone to Choleric disorders, following a cooling, anti-Choleric dietary regimen will go a long way towards preventing or mitigating the occurrence of acute or serious Choleric flare-ups.

The first thing we must do is to eliminate those foods which cause or aggravate Choleric excess or disorder. These are mainly fried foods, greasy foods, excessive salt, excessive aged cheeses, excessive red meat and animal fats, and excessive alcohol and spicy foods.

Coffee, although it may be bitter, is not therapeutic, but actually injurious to the liver and bile metabolism; in addition, the stimulant effects of its caffeine fire up the nerves, and can cause Choleric aggravations of the nervous system. Also, coffee is grown mainly in tropical third world countries, which use a lot of pesticides in growing it, which are toxic to the liver.

The anti-Choleric diet contains a great abundance of fresh fruits and vegetables to alkalize cool and detoxify the blood. Of these, certain ones are particularly beneficial and therapeutic.

Adjusting and regulating black bile

Black Bile, also called Melancholy or Atrabile, is the humor that is most prone to aggravations and pathology; more pathological conditions are attributable to disorders of Black Bile than to any other humor. The reasons for this are two-fold:

• Under normal, healthy conditions, Black Bile's optimum level or proportion in the human body is less than that for any other humor, making it the humor most inherently prone to excess and aggravation.
• Blood is the humor most essential and conducive to vitality and good health; Black Bile is contrary to Blood in all its qualities and attributes, making it the humor most prone to pathology and disease.

In addition, Black Bile, of all the Four Humors, takes the longest time to ripen, or be concocted so that superfluities of it may be purged or expelled, being in this attribute as well contrary to Blood, or the Sanguine humor. Black Bile takes at least fifteen days to ripen, so a course of therapy to adjust or correct imbalances of Black Bile must be followed for at least fifteen days before any definite positive changes can be seen.

The Manifestations of Black Bile Imbalance

The pathological manifestations of Black Bile imbalance are indeed many and varied, and can affect virtually any organ or part of the body. Because the pathological manifestations of Black Bile imbalance are so many and varied, an equal diversity of therapeutic modalities, strategies and approaches are needed to correct them.

In the brain, mind and nervous system, also called the Psychic Faculty in Persian Medicine, troubles and afflictions are usually due to the subtler, vaporous forms of Black Bile, also called Melancholy or the Nervous humor, rising up to the head and brain. The deleterious effects of aggravated Black Bile are seen as nervousness, giddiness or lightheadedness, tinnitus or ringing in the ears, neurasthenia or nervous exhaustion, tremors, tics and spasms. And so, the herbs and therapies used to treat these conditions have sedative, nervine, antispasmodic and antidepressant effects.

In the musculoskeletal system, aggravated Black Bile will cause arthritic and rheumatic disorders characterized by dryness, hardness, stiffness, tension, and asthenia, or wasting. These are treated with antirheumatics, vulneraries and antispasmodics. Neuromuscular disorders are also usually due to aggravated Black Bile, and are characterized by wasting, numbness, tremors, spasms, and asthenia; these are treated with the appropriate antispasmodics, nervous tonics and restoratives.

It must be remembered here that conditions of ischemia, or deficient blood supply to the muscles and tissues, joints and tendons is in fact a Melancholic condition, because the absence of Hot, moistening Blood will produce a cold, dry Melancholic condition. And so, increasing the circulation and vital blood supply to an organ or tissue of the body is actually an anti-Melancholic therapeutic approach.

In the respiratory tract, Melancholic conditions arise or are aggravated by the cold, dry weather that prevails in the fall, which can cause dryness, thirst and fits of spasmodic coughing. These are remedied with the appropriate antitussives and antispasmodics, as well as moistening, soothing demulcents and emollients.

In the liver and hepatobiliary system, aggravations of Black Bile can cause hepatobiliary insufficiency and other asthenic and cirrhotic conditions of the liver, biliary dyskinesia and calculi, and poor blood circulation, hypertension and stagnation in the hepatic portal system. These conditions are treated with the appropriate cholagogues, hepatobiliary tonics and Black Bile purgatives. Aggravated Black Bile in the liver will also cause pain, distension and discomfort under the lower ribs, or hypochondriac region, a condition generally referred to as Melancholia.

Since the spleen is the storage receptacle for Black Bile, this organ is especially vulnerable to excesses and aggravations of that humor, which can cause conditions of indigestion, anorexia or poor appetite, irritable bowel or intestinal obstruction. These conditions are treated with Splenicals, which remove obstructions and morbidity from the spleen.

In the GI tract, aggravations of Black Bile result in poor appetite, indigestion, sour stomach, epigastric or abdominal colic, distension, gas or bloating, irritable bowel and constipation. Generally, these disorders are treated with herbs and medicines that are cholagogue, stomachic, carminative, laxative and aperient; although herbs in these categories are numerous, there are certain special herbs that are particularly adept at adjusting and regulating disorders of Black Bile in cases in which this humor is the cause. Excessively harsh or astringent herbs tend to aggravate Black Bile in the GI tract, whereas soothing, moistening demulcents and emollients relieve it.

In the skin, aggravated Black Bile causes chronic skin conditions, usually characterized by itching, dryness and scaling. Scales and lesions which are surrounded by bright pink, but in which the scale or scab is a milky white are usually caused by Black Bile. Alternatives that cleanse morbid Black Bile from the blood and lymph are used to treat these conditions.

Fevers caused by a putrefaction of morbid Black Bile are called intermittent fevers that come on every fourth day. They are treated with the appropriate antiperiodics.

Since Black Bile is cold and dry in temperament, herbs and therapies used to subdue or eliminate aggravated Black Bile tend to be Hot and moistening in nature. Pungent and bitter herbs work well in stimulating the metabolism and ripening of Black Bile, and dispersing its blockages. Many herbs that treat aggravations of Black Bile also seem to have a musky or earthy aroma to them, which resonates with the humor's associated Earth element.

Black Bile and Cancer

In Persian Medicine, morbid Black Bile was considered to be the humor most implicated in cancer. This is because cancerous tumors, in their gross, manifest properties and appearance, have qualities commonly associated with Black Bile and the Earth element: they are hard, cold, dark in color, and firmly rooted or embedded in the surrounding tissue.

Conventional allopathic medicine sees the cancerous growth or tumor as a pathogenic invader, as a group of mutant renegade cells trying to take over an otherwise normal host. And so, its main therapies have been focused on trying to cut burn or poison these mutant cells out of the body.

But this approach is quite myopic and shortsighted, and yields only limited success. The radical intervention of conventional cancer treatment can be very debilitating to the host organism as a whole; if the patient recovers, it is too often in spite of the treatment, not because of it. The holistic approach of Persian Medicine and other natural healing systems is to see the malignant growth as merely the surface manifestation of a deeper systemic malignancy or derangement. In order for recovery from cancer to be lasting or complete, these deeper disorders must be addressed.

Although morbid, oxidized forms of Black Bile are involved in the process of carcinogenesis, in cancer, the whole metabolism, and all of the humors, is deranged. This profound morbidity and derangement of all the humors is evidenced by the sickly, cachexic complexion of so many cancer patients, particularly in the advanced stages of the disease.

To put the metabolism back in order, pepsis and the Digestive Fire must be stimulationd. The liver, which generates and regulates all the humors, must be thoroughly cleansed, its temperament rectified, and its humoral metabolism normalized. The functions of all the eliminative organs, especially the liver and the colon, must be greatly stimulationd to evacuate accumulated metabolic wastes. The blood, spleen and lymphatic system must be cleansed with herbal blood cleansers, or alteratives.

Cancer also involves a profound derangement and depletion of the immune system. Even in the normal, healthy person, stray mutant cancer cells are generated from time to time, but the host's immune system destroys these abnormal cells before they can take root, grow and metastasize. But by the time cancer finally takes hold, the host's immune system is already greatly compromised.

Malignant tumors often form in areas where the flow of blood has become compromised, congested or stagnant. According to Persian Medicine, the stagnant blood purifies and mixes with morbid charred or oxidized forms of Black Bile, forming the hard nodule of a tumor. The fact that putrefactive processes are involved is evident from the fact that, when a cancerous tumor is incised or cut open, a foul, putrid odor issues forth.

The Phlegmatic humor, especially the lymph, provides an important supporting role in maintaining optimum immunity. If the lymphatic system does not purify the lymph, plasma and serous fluids, which are recycled back into the bloodstream, immunity will suffer. And the spleen, the largest lymphatic organ in the body, depends on the Retentive Virtue and chelating action of the normal Black Bile it stores to filter particulate impurities out of the blood and lymph.

When fighting a chronic degenerative disease like cancer by natural means, a comprehensive treatment plan must be devised, preferably under the guidance of a holistic healthcare professional. Such a treatment regimen must incorporate the following:

Dietary Therapy, since diet profoundly affects our metabolism, as well as the humoral balance and purity of the organism.

Herbal Therapy to cleanse the liver and bowels, blood and lymph, to stimulation and balance pepsis and metabolism, dissolve tumors, nodules and accumulations of morbid humors, and to support and stimulation the immune response of the organism.

Hygienic Purification Therapies like colonics and enemas to remove accumulated waste matter from the body.

Nutritional Supplementation to give the body the vital nutrients it needs for optimum constitutional strength and resilience to fight the cancer and win. Lifestyle and Psychological Therapy to ensure adequate exercise and rest, constructive living habits, and a positive mental and emotional outlook, which benefits the overall immunity of the body and strengthens the will to live.

With natural methods as well as conventional, early, prompt diagnosis and treatment are all important. Our chances for total victory against the cancer are much better if we catch it while it is still a localized phenomenon; after the cancer metastasizes and spreads systemically; our chances for recovery get a lot slimmer.

Understanding the healing crisis

Due to the many pathogenic influences and stresses of daily life, as well as environmental toxicity and pollution, and the various imbalances and defects that can crop up in the process of pepsis, or digestion and metabolism, toxins, metabolic wastes, and morbid or superfluous humors inevitably accumulate in the organism over time. If the body is to remain strong, vital and healthy, it must be periodically cleansed and detoxified.

If the body's eliminative organs are not functioning optimally in the cleansing and detoxification of the organism, and they often aren't, there will be some residual or remedial cleansing and detoxification work that needs to be done. This is done through certain hygienic purification therapies, or what Avicenna called procured evacuations, in which the physician provokes certain cleansing or detoxifying responses from the organism to eliminate the offending toxins and waste.

The Six Hygienic Purification Therapies of Persian Medicine are diaphoresis, diuresis, emesis, purgation, venesection and derivation. They provoke the natural cleansing and detoxification responses of the organism, and utilize all the major eliminative organs and channels of the body, as follows:

Diaphoresis: Sweating - Skin

Diuresis: Urination - Kidneys and Urinary Tract

Emesis: Vomiting - Lungs, Stomach, Upper GI Tract

Purgation: Stool - Bowels

Venesection: Bleeding - Veins and Blood

Derivation: Flushing, Blisters and Boils - Skin

But it's important to remember that all these Hygienic Purification Therapies, or procured evacuations, are remedial in nature, to be used only to relieve certain toxic conditions and toxicity signs and symptoms, as indicated. They were designed to provoke cleansing responses from the organism that are in imitation of the natural, spontaneous cleansing processes and reactions of the body.

Ideally, the body and its eliminative organs should be doing for itself what these various Hygienic Purification Therapies are provoking the organism to do. And when conditions are right, and when the inherent vital forces of the organism are sufficiently strong, balanced and robust, the organism will spontaneously eliminate accumulated wastes and toxins by the most appropriate, accessible and convenient route open to it. When such spontaneous cleansing and regeneration on the part of the organism gets particularly acute and dramatic, it is called a Healing Crisis.

The various cleansing reactions that may be experienced during a Healing Crisis, and the particular Hygienic Purification Therapies that imitate or provoke these reactions, are as follows:

- The body may sweat excessively or dramatically (Diaphoresis).
- There may be vigorous or dramatic elimination through the urine (Diuresis).
- There may be spontaneous nausea, giddiness, regurgitation or vomiting (Emesis).
- There may be acute, spontaneous episodes of loose stools or diarrhea (Purgation).
- There may be spontaneous bleeding, as in nosebleeds (Venesection or Bloodletting).

There may be spontaneous flushing or changing of the complexion, or the formation of blisters, pustules or boils to eliminate accumulated pus, toxins and morbid or superfluous humors (Derivation).

When it comes to the Healing Crisis, there's a huge philosophical difference between conventional allopathic medicine and Persian Medicine. Modern allopathic medicine sees these signs of the Healing Crisis as troublesome reactions that must be covered up or suppressed, whereas Persian Medicine welcomes them as great opportunities for healing, detoxification and recovery. The only catch is that the physician has to clinically be able to tell the difference between signs heralding a genuine Healing Crisis and the onset of disease symptoms.

Palliation versus Healing

Palliation is doing the most convenient and expedient thing to get rid of the surface symptoms of the disorder as quickly as possible. Healing is removing or resolving all aspects of the disorder, both latent and manifest, by treating its root cause.

Palliation is too often a mere stopgap measure, a way of putting off having to really heal and resolve the disorder until later. Palliation, especially in modern medicine, all too frequently means simply masking or suppressing the surface symptoms, which usually drives the disorder deeper within the organism, to resurface later in a more serious form. Pharmaceutical drugs that mask the symptoms create many undesirable side effects, which are signs that the organism is protesting as the underlying disease or disorder is driven deeper.

Nevertheless, there may be certain situations, even when using natural healing methods, in which palliation may be the wisest and best way of dealing with an acute crisis situation. If a fire is raging out of control, first put out the fire, because that's the most urgent order of business, and then rebuild the house.

Unfortunately, too much of modern medicine is mere palliation, as disease and crisis management, and too little of it is true healing. To modern medicine, true healing may be a lost art, impatiently shoved aside in our search for magic bullets and quick fixes. True healing always takes time, and comes in its own sweet time if we strive to improve our overall state of health.

The true physician and natural healer must work on two levels to provide his patient with complete and comprehensive healthcare. On the surface, he is giving the patient palliative measures, as necessary, to get him safely through temporary health difficulties and/or crisis situations. But beyond this, on a deeper level, he is always seeking to guide the patient towards a greater level of overall health, balance and wellbeing, in which his innate vitality and resistance would be able to adequately support and manifest a Healing Crisis.

Signs of the Healing Crisis

The whole gist of the Healing Crisis is this: If you have undertaken a program to detoxify and truly restore your health, that you may experience a temporary period of feeling worse before you finally feel better. The strange thing is that these distressing signs and symptoms of the Healing Crisis may suddenly come on just after you feel that you've achieved a new, higher level of overall health, balance and wellbeing.

The path back to better health is not a straight, linear progression; neither is it all a bed of roses. Nevertheless, the onset of the Healing Crisis should be welcomed with joy and gladness, because the organism, no longer burdened with having to cope with disease symptoms and morbidity on a constant, daily basis, can now turn its energies and resources towards true healing and regeneration, and the throwing off of old, latent problems and conditions that may be holding it back.

Whatever the particular signs and symptoms of the Healing Crisis may be, there are three crucial differences that distinguish the Healing Crisis from the onset of disease symptoms:

• Core energy and vitality levels are good and improving; with disease onset, there is oppression and devitalization.

• Signs and symptoms of a true Healing Crisis are much more temporary and transient, lasting only days instead of weeks, months or even years.
• The general progression and enfoldment of signs and symptoms in the

Hakim G. M. Chishti in The Healer's Handbook tells us what preliminary signs and symptoms presage the onset of various forms of spontaneous elimination and detoxification during the Healing Crisis, so that we may have an idea of what is to come. If the elimination and detoxification crisis episode is to happen during the day, these preliminary signs and symptoms will appear the previous night, and if the acute episode is to happen during the night, they will appear on the previous day.

Crisis by vomiting: wheezing or dyspnea, a change in the breathing rhythm, a bitter taste in the mouth, pain in the cardia or upper epigastrium, stomach convulsions, a lowered pulse and trembling of the lower lip.

Crisis by diarrhea: intestinal pain and cramping, heaviness of the body, stomach gas, backache, strangely colored or formed stools, and grumbling intestines.

Crisis by nosebleed: dull sense of hearing, ringing in the ears, tears, nose itching, and a full pulse in the arteries of the temples.

Crisis by urination: heaviness and distension in the bladder, thick excessive urine, and bright urine color on the fourth day of a detoxification program, and the actual crisis on the seventh day.

Crisis by sweating: lightheadedness, itching, alternating chills and feverishness.

Although a Healing Crisis can come on totally spontaneously, this is not often the case. It is usually earned by undergoing a program of cleansing, detoxification and health improvement.

And neither is the Healing Crisis, once experienced and gone through, a magic silver bullet or a permanent and final solution to all one's health problems. The process of healing and regeneration occurs in growth spurts and plateaus; the growth spurts are the Healing Crises, when the organism is struggling to achieve a new level of health and regeneration, whereas the plateaus are settling in periods in which the organism stabilizes and accustoms itself to operating on a new level.

Therapeutic Management of the Healing Crisis

Once the Healing Crisis starts, whatever form it takes, the most important thing a physician or healer can do is to stay out of the way and not interfere, as much as possible. Do not step in and interfere with the crucial elimination, detoxification, healing and regeneration that the body is trying to do for itself. Above all, palliative measures that merely suppress or mask the symptoms without getting to the root of the problem must be avoided. They will usually stop the Healing Crisis dead in its tracks.

Neither should one second guess what the body is going to do at the onset of a Healing Crisis, and then give remedies, even natural ones, to help the process along. This will only confuse and/or weaken the natural cleansing and healing reactions of the organism, especially if you predicted wrongly.

For example, it may appear, from all preliminary signs, that crisis by vomiting is imminent. But in some cases, what may initially seem like an impending crisis by vomiting may turn to diarrhea at the last moment. If you had prognosticated that crisis by vomiting was definitely in the works and had given an emetic to help it along, you would have only wound up confusing the natural cleansing reactions and innate healing wisdom of the organism. Even if your prognostication had been right, and the organism was indeed headed for crisis by vomiting, the emetic would have only weakened the body's natural cleansing reactions, and substituted an artificial aid or crutch for the real Healing Crisis.

Dietary, the physician or therapist should not interfere with the cleansing and purification the organism is trying to accomplish during the Healing Crisis by burdening it with a lot of heavy or hard to digest foods. This will also stop the Healing Crisis dead in its tracks.

Generally speaking, the more intense and vehement the symptoms of the Healing Crisis are, especially the gastrointestinal symptoms, the lighter and more restricted should be the diet. And when the crisis is in the acute phase and the signs and symptoms are at their most intense, only a liquid diet should be administered, such as diluted fresh fruit or vegetable juices, herb teas or vegetable broths.

Until the acute phase of the Healing Crisis comes, a light and easily digestible diet that provides basic caloric energy and nutrient, mineral and electrolyte support should be given. In designing the appropriate dietary regimen, two basic factors must be taken into consideration:

1) The closeness or imminence of the acute phase of the Healing Crisis;

2) The constitutional needs of the patient as to what kind of diet he or she can support.

The closer or more imminent the acute phase of the Healing Crisis gets, the lighter and more restricted should be the diet until, at the acute phase, only a liquid diet should be given. While in the preparatory and recovery phases before and after the acute phase, a light diet of vegetable soups and stews, or barley gruel, also known as ptisan, may be given.

Constitutionally, more robust individuals are able to withstand a lighter, more restricted diet and still manage to maintain their basic strength and vitality. Those whose constitution is more frail and delicate need a heartier, more nutritious diet in the preparatory phase to give them the basic vitality needed to withstand the cleansing and detoxification.

The herbal teas used during the Healing Crisis, especially in its acute phase, should be gentle and mild, and support the organism in the cleansing it is trying to accomplish.

During the acute phase of the Healing Crisis, no alteration or innovation should be made in the treatment or the regimen. Rather, things should be kept the same, so as not to impose any undue Stimulation or shocks on the organism, and let it do its healing and cleansing work undisturbed.

Therapeutic foods

Food is Your Best Medicine

Avicenna said, "Let your food be your medicine, and your medicine be your food." There's essentially no difference between food and medicine. The difference between food and medicine isn't one of kind; it's merely one of degree.

Foods have the same kinds of therapeutic properties that herbs and medicines have; it's just that in foods, these therapeutic properties are milder in degree, whereas the nutritive properties are stronger. Herbs and natural medicines have more potent and concentrated therapeutic properties, but they also have nutritive value, which synthetic pharmaceutical drugs lack. If foods are essentially like medicines in having therapeutic properties, it follows that many, in addition to having indications, or conditions that they're used for, have contra-indications as well, or conditions in which they do harm, and should not be taken.

This kind of therapeutic knowledge of the indications and contraindications of various foods is a common feature and legacy of Persian Medicine and other healing systems. This is a practical, empirical knowledge derived from centuries of clinical experience. It concerns the basic qualities and properties of foods, and is not based upon a food's nutrient content.

Making and Taking Herbal Medicines

Herbal medicines, in various forms, were personally formulated and compounded, as directed by the patient's physician. Simple raw ingredients and/or pre-formulated standard preparations were mixed together in the right proportions, and in the right form, to produce the desired effect. Not only the herbs or medicines you take, but their dosage, form of preparation, and mode of administration are important to maximize the medicine's effectiveness.

Simples versus Formulas

A tea or other preparation made from just one herb is called a simple. A medicinal preparation containing two or more ingredients is called a formula.

Whenever possible, keep it simple; if just one herb meets all your needs, take that herb alone as a simple. If no single herb alone meets all your needs, you may have to take a formula. Even here, keep it simple; the simplest formula that addresses all your needs is usually the best. When in doubt, it's best to use an established classical formula according to its indications.

Making an effective herbal formula is a sophisticated art as well as a science. There's much more involved in making an herbal formula than just the crude "shotgun approach" of putting together every herb you know of that treats the ailment under consideration. Ly, herbs were selected according to their basic actions, tastes and energetics so that they worked harmoniously together.

Persian Medicine at a glance

Introduction and concepts

Summary

The Persian doctrine of Medicine is a comprehensive medical system, which meticulously deals with the various states of health and disease. It provides promotive, preventive, curative and rehabilitative healthcare. The fundamentals, diagnosis and treatment modalities of the system are based on scientific principles and holistic concepts of health and healing. Its holistic approach considers individual in relation to his environment and stresses on health of body, mind and soul. Temperament of a patient is given great importance in diagnosis and treatment of diseases with natural remedies derived mostly from plants. Temperament is also taken into consideration for identifying the most suitable diet and lifestyle for promoting the health of a particular individual.

The Persian doctrine of Medicine considers the entire universe including human being, disease, drugs, environmental factors etc. to be intrinsically defined by four primary Qualities - Hot: Cold and Dry: Wet. These Qualities are reflected in all the basic concepts of Persian doctrine of Medicine such as Elements, Temperament, Humors etc. which are used for describing and correlating human health and disease with promotive and curative factors e.g. diet, drugs etc. Persian doctrine of Medicine prescribes a methodology to infer a treatment on the basis of Temperament and to test it experimentally during the course of treatment. This accounts for the clinical reproducibility of the therapeutic effects of Persian Medicine treatment.

The Persian doctrine of Medicine diagnoses and treats the patient as a whole looking into their overall physical, mental and spiritual aspects. The therapeutics in Persian doctrine of Medicine is described under the major headings of Regimental therapy,

Dietotherapy, Pharmacotherapy and Surgery. Regimental therapy along with Dietotherapy is considered the best approach for promotion of health and treatment of disease. Persian doctrine of Medicine has also emphasized the importance of psychiatric treatment in the management of various diseases. Surgical interventions and procedures are elaborately described and practiced in conditions, which are not amenable to drug treatment. (67-68)

History of Persian Medicine

Among the great medical traditions of the world, traditional Iranian medicine has left an indelible imprint upon the practice of healing.

Among the many notable examples of important Iranian contributors to medicine include the philosopher-scientist Ibn Sina (Avicenna, c. 980 – 1037 C.E.), whose text "Canon of Medicine" was in use by physicians all over the western and middle-eastern world for over 600 years.

Razi (Rhazes)

Initially it was the school of medicine in Jundishapur that inspired the early Muslim physicians, with an emphasis upon rational inquiry, and preventative regimens such as diet and exercise. Perhaps no other Islamic physician best exemplified this approach than Abu Bakr Muhammad ibn Zakariya' al-Razi (c. 865 – 925 C.E.), who stated "where a cure can be obtained by diet, use no drugs and avoid complex remedies where simple ones will suffice." Razi, later known to the European world as "Rhazes," was a brilliant clinician, musician, philosopher, and alchemist. One story recounts that al Razi determined the location for a hospital in Baghdad after setting out raw meat in four different quarters of the city. The meat located in the quarter of the city that had undergone the smallest degree of putrefaction was then chosen as the location for the new hospital.

Among his many contributions to medical science, the Kitab al-Hawi fi al-tibb (Comprehensive Book on Medicine) has been revered by physicians for centuries, both in the Muslim world and in Europe.

Razi appears to have been a pragmatic physician, emphasizing his interest in therapeutics as opposed to theory and the classification of symptoms. He certainly relied upon the work of Galen, but was not so in awe of him that he wouldn't correct what he perceived to be errors. For example, Razi said that the many cases of fever he observed in the hospitals of Baghdad did not conform to Galen's description. Razi maintained a flexible and inspired approach to healing, but was not interested in altering the theoretical foundations of Hippocrates or Galen.

Ibn Sina (Avicenna)

The pragmatic and flexible emphasis of al Razi however, was eventually superseded by the intellectual rigor of Abu `Ali al Husayn ibn `Abd Allah ibn Sina, or more simply, Ibn Sina (Avicenna, c. 980 – 1037 C.E.), considered by many to be the greatest of the Iranian scientists. Ibn Sina was born in 980 C.E. Ibn Sina demonstrated his genius at an early age, memorizing the holy Qur'an by the age of 10, and beginning his studies in medicine when he was only 17, pronouncing that the subject was, in his own words, "not difficult". By the age of 18 Ibn Sina had built up a reputation as an excellent physician.

To friends that were concerned for him and suggested he slow down, Ibn Sina said "I prefer a short life with width to a narrow one with length".

Beyond his consummate devotion to his work and his genius for retaining information, Ibn Sina shared with Galen a passion for order, to arrange facts and phenomena into a coherent system of knowledge. Among his scientific works, the most important are the Kitab al Shifa (Book of Healing), a philosophical encyclopedia based upon Aristotelian philosophy, and the million-word al Qanun fi al Tibb (Canon of Medicine), representing the "final codification of Iranian" concepts on medicine. The Qanun is divided into five books, the first dealing with general principles of medicine; the second with simple plant drugs arranged in alphabetical order; the third with diseases of particular organs and tissues of the body; the fourth with local diseases that spread to other parts of the body, such as fever; and the fifth with complex formulae. Ibn Sina demonstrates his many clinical insights in the Qanun, detailing for example the contagious nature of tuberculosis and its spread by soil and water. He provides a differential diagnosis of ancylostomiasis (hookworm disease) and attributes the condition to an intestinal worm (Monzur 1990; Savage-Smith 1994). The Qanun's materia medica details some 760 drugs, commenting on their usage and efficacy. In this text, Ibn Sina was also among the first to recommend the testing of a new drug on animals and humans before their widespread usage. To his contemporaries, Ibn Sina's al-Qanun was the perfection of medicine, displaying an almost mathematical accuracy that ensured its unrivaled status as the most important text of Persian Medicine. But lest we content ourselves by defining Ibn Sina as a man of medicine, we should not forget his authority on a wide variety of subjects including philosophy, theology, geometry, and astrology.

Introduction

The Persian doctrine of Medicine is a medical system that deals with the management of health and diseases. It provides preventive, promotive, curative and rehabilitative healthcare with holistic approach. The fundamental framework of this system is based on deep philosophical insights and scientific principles, including the theory of four Elements I.e. Air, Water, Fire and Earth; four proximate Qualities I.e. Hot, Cold, Wet and Dry, and the theory of four Humors; Blood, Phlegm, Yellow Bile and Black Bile. Admixture of different Elements and their Qualities in specific ratio in a particular entity, whether living or non-living, denominates its Temperament. Human Temperament is commonly denoted by the dominant Humor I.e. Sanguine, Phlegmatic, Choleric and Melancholic, which can be correlated with the Temperament of Diet, Drugs, Environmental Factors etc. as the entities of non-human Universe being made up directly of Elements are described in terms of Qualitative Temperament. Any disturbance in the equilibrium of Humors causes disease, and therefore the treatment aims at restoring the equilibrium by giving factors (including drugs) of opposite temperament. In addition, Persian doctrine of Medicine believes that Medicatrix natura is the supreme power, which controls all the physiological functions of the body, provides resistance against the diseases and helps in healing naturally.

The Persian doctrine of Medicine is holistic in nature and takes into account the whole personality rather than taking a reductionist approach towards disease. Persian Medicine physicians give prime importance to diet and the state of digestion in a person, in both health and disease. Specific dietary regimens are recommended while treating patients according to their temperament. Proper diets are assumed to produce good Humors while improper ones produce bad Humors. Thus, the humoral imbalance can be corrected by medication coupled with proper diet. The physician prescribes the drugs according to the temperament of patient, causative Humor, faculty of organ involved and severity of the disease. These drugs are classified as per the specific temperament and are graded in the first, second, third and fourth degree according to their potency.

The Persian doctrine of Medicine offers treatment of diseases related to all the systems and organs of the human body. The treatments for chronic ailments and diseases of skin, liver, musculo-skeletal and reproductive systems, immunological and lifestyle disorders have been found to be highly effective and acceptable. The use of elative, exhilarants, aphrodisiacs, organ-specific tonics and immuno-modulatory drugs, temperament specific drugs, correctives for adverse effects, concoctive and purgatives etc. are unique features of Persian doctrine of Medicine.

Despite vast development in the field of modern medicine and surgery, there is a growing global interest in traditional systems of medicine.

Strengths of Persian doctrine of medicine

The basic strengths of Persian doctrine of Medicine are its

holistic approach, temperament based prescription and treatment. The use of natural drugs (mainly of plant origin), various therapeutic interventions, and regimens for prevention and treatment of diseases and health promotion is based on the concepts of holistic healing considering the individual's psycho-physical wellbeing. Rational use of Persian Medicine medicines is usually free from adverse effects. The toning up of the organs and the immune system is a unique approach of Persian Medicine known for its beneficial effects. In chronic and some of the intractable diseases, these approaches have shown much utility in improving the quality of life of patients.

Unique concept of Temperament: Persian doctrine of Medicine believes that every individual has its own unique temperament according to their humoral constitution, lifestyle and environment. Any deviation from its normal temperament results into disease. The management of the disease depends upon the correction of altered temperament by using various regimens and drugs.

Holistic approach: For the management of a disease, Persian doctrine of Medicine takes entire constitution of the individual and lifestyle into account for diagnosing and prescribing the treatment. Physicians select the drugs and regimens according to the temperament of the patient and nature of the disease.

Safe and radical cure of chronic ailments: The thrust area of Persian doctrine of Medicine is the management of chronic diseases. It provides radical and safe cure for various chronic disorders, such as psychoneurotic disorders, hepato-biliary disorders, gastro-intestinal disorders, metabolic disorders etc.

Prevention of disease and promotion of health: Apart from treating disease conditions, Persian doctrine of Medicine lays great emphasis on the prevention of disease and promotion of existing health through principles of six essential factors of life.

Regimental therapy: Persian doctrine of Medicine makes use of certain special modes and regimens of diet, physical movements, lifestyle etc. and techniques such as cupping, leeching, venesection etc. to eliminate the morbid Humors from the body.

Immunomodulation: Persian doctrine of Medicine believes that the real physician is the body's intrinsic power of healing and maintaining its normal state of health. Accordingly, a number of drugs are available which boost up the immunity of the body. In diseases like Tuberculosis, AIDS, Cancer etc. where the long-term therapy is required, the Persian Medicine drugs, used as adjuvant, play an important role in reducing the toxicity of the synthetic drugs and in modulating or enhancing the body immunity and improving the overall quality of life.

Tonics: The concept of using organ- and system-specific tonics is a unique feature of Persian doctrine of Medicine. Iranian physicians have described a number of drugs to strengthen and tone up various vital organs of the body. The literature is replete with a number of these formulations such as Cardiac Tonics, Nervine Tonics, Liver Tonics and Kidney Tonics. Tonics improving digestive power are also used in chronic gastrointestinal disorders.

Exhilarants: This is a special group of drugs which creates feeling of happiness by relaxing the mind and heart from various stresses. This group of drugs is used in the management of neuropsychiatric and cardiac disorders e.g. Anxiety, Depression, Palpitation etc. These drugs also create an overall feeling of wellbeing, which is a uniqueness of Persian doctrine of Medicine.

Specialties: Persian doctrine of Medicine offers successful treatment for various diseases especially the chronic ones. These include skin diseases like Vitiligo, Eczema, Psoriasis etc.; Digestive disorders e.g. Acid peptic disease, dyspepsia, Irritable Bowel Syndrome (IBS), Ulcerative colitis etc.; Respiratory disorders such as Bronchial asthma, Chronic bronchitis etc.; Musculo-skeletal disorders e.g. Arthritis and Osteoporosis; Neurological disorders e.g. Senile dementia, Paresis, Paralysis etc.; Cardio-vascular disorders such as Hypertension, Ischemic heart disease etc.; Lifestyle and Metabolic disorders e.g. Obesity, Hyperlipidemia, Gout, Diabetes mellitus etc. and Sexual disorders e.g. Erectile dysfunction, Premature ejaculation, Loss of libido etc.

Global scenario

WHO efforts and strategies for strengthening primary healthcare have played an instrumental role in the development of traditional medicine across the globe. With Alma Ata declaration of 1978 to achieve the goal of 'Health for All' involving medicine and its practitioners in primary healthcare delivery, policies and strategic interventions were designed to facilitate peoples, access to healthcare through medicine, and WHO supported these initiatives in member countries with publication of technical documents and guidelines. A number of World Health Assembly resolutions are aimed at scientific development of traditional medicine and medicinal plants for their best use in the healthcare of the populations. These developments equally impacted Persian doctrine of Medicine. Persian doctrine is popular in different parts of the world with different names.

Fundamentals of Persian doctrine of medicine

The unique holistic approach and clinical success of the Persian doctrine of Medicine arise from its Fundamental Principles. The most important of these principles is Temperament which classifies human beings, diet, drugs etc. into Four Qualitative Types: Hot & Dry, Hot & Wet, Cold & Wet and Cold & Dry. There are different sets of observable parameters for identifying the qualitative Temperament in human beings, diets and drugs etc. The Temperament of a man is found by certain bodily and mental characters, for instance a Hot & Dry Temperament is associated with a lean built, excessive anger etc. The Temperament of diet, drug etc. is known by some physical characters and effects on human beings, for example, a non-succulent, pungent or salty vegetable is likely to be Hot & Dry. This allows the identification of the diet which is proper for maintaining the healthy Temperament of a human being, e.g. a person having Hot & Dry temperament should use more of a moderately Hot & Dry diet to maintain his normal temperament and remain healthy. However Persian doctrine of Medicine clearly mentions that the appropriate diet thus inferred should be actually tried in man and shown to maintain health before being accepted. Thus, it uses its principles only for hypothesizing an effect which has to be confirmed by experimental testing.

Disease is characterized by a pathological shift in Temperament, e.g. a Hot & Dry man becoming abnormally Cold & Wet may start suffering from severe arthritis. Using only pain-killers will just give symptomatic relief and may have side-effects. By reversing the abnormal Cold & Wet Temperament to the normal Hot & Dry one by using a Hot & Dry drug will cure his arthritis safely.

Treatment on the basis of Temperament has been found to be actually effective in diverse regions. Molecular level Pharmacological Testing has revealed molecular mechanisms behind the clinical effects of Persian Medicine Drugs. So it becomes quite evident that Temperament and other Fundamental Principles discovered in Persian doctrine of Medicine reflect biological and physico-chemical reality.

The Persian doctrine of Medicine possesses fundamental principles for all medical fields i.e. Physiology Preventive Medicine, Pathology, Diagnostics, Pharmacology and Therapeutics. The principles related to human biology are the seven Natural Factors that make up the totality of a human being, viz. Elements, Humors, Temperament, Organs, Pneuma, Faculties and Functions. The imbalance in the Temperament and Humors, disorganization and discontinuity of the structure leads to the development of disease. The Persian doctrine of Medicine uses macroscopic parameters to diagnose the disease which comprise of clinical history, physical examination, Pulse examination and inspection of excreta. The concept of treatment is based upon the removal of the causative factor, evacuation of morbid material and normalization of the morbid temperament. This is achieved as per the principles of Heterotherapy, by using the drugs and diets of opposite temperament, i.e. Drug Treatment and Dietary Treatment, respectively Non-drug manipulative techniques or regimens like Bath, Massage, and Leeching etc. Surgery, Psychiatric Treatment and Spiritual Treatment are also used.

The Persian doctrine of Medicine enjoins Preventive Medicine, or what it calls positively as Maintenance of Health to be more important than Treatment. This is divided into three parts: Maintenance of Health, as such, Regimens for Debility and Prevention of Disease. In a completely healthy person it prescribes a lifestyle, diet and environment, appropriate for his or her Temperament, while in healthy but weak persons or healthy persons, who have become vulnerable to disease, special diets, non-drug manipulative techniques s or regimens and even drugs are prescribed to maintain health and prevent disease.

Development of concepts

There is a long history of the development of fundamental concepts in Persian doctrine of Medicine which emerged due to the contribution and interaction of culturally and intellectually diverse civilizations. First the idea of a basic character of human being, drugs etc. or 'temperament' emerged. After is introduced the empirically apprehensible four basic Qualities: Hot: Cold and Dry: Wet, as the indicators of the basic and holistic character of 'temperament'. The Qualities were posited to exist in the Four Elements described. The Iranian Hakims were devoted to unity and objectivity. So, on the one hand, they systematized all aspects of physiology, pathology, pharmacology, environmental influences etc. on the basis of the common and simple scheme of Hot: Cold & Dry: Wet in a fully integrated system without any gaps. This was perfected in Ibn Sina's the Canon of Medicine. On the other hand, they made rigorous observations and experimentation. The resulting clinical and therapeutic observations are most comprehensively recorded by Razi in his gigantic work of 23 volumes, namely, Al-Hawi. The Persian doctrine of Medicine gave great importance to the Humoral Theory to emphasize the unique character of Living Things/Organic Matter and their distinction from Non-living Things/Inorganic Matter by explaining that the Elements are metabolized and converted into Humors, which are organic and possess the additional properties of living things. It describes four

Humors and says that the Temperament of human beings depends upon the dominant Humor. However, since each Humor possesses particular Qualities, it is possible to convert Humoral Temperament into Qualitative Temperament and then easily correlate human states with Drugs, Diets etc., which are described directly by Qualitative Temperament. The Iranian scholars provided a strong basis for the correlation of the Humoral Theory with scientific Clinical Studies by discovering the Clinical Parameters of Humors which they called as Ten Categories. The Iranians took the Pharmacology based upon the Qualitative Temperament of Drugs but they brought in Observation by discovering the physical parameters of Qualitative Temperament. They tremendously increased the role of observation and experimentation by proposing that Drugs act not only by Qualities but also by their Essence and since, unlike Qualities, the Essence cannot be known by physical parameters, the Pharmacological Actions arising from Essence can be discovered only by random empirical observation.

Basic principles

The Persian doctrine of Medicine is successful in providing holistic treatment i.e. Radical cure without significant adverse effects. Further, it is very easy to practice and always produces the reported effects. The majority of clinical trials on Persian Medicine treatment have found them to be effective. Drugs hypothesized to be effective in new diseases on the basis of Persian Medicine principles have been found to actually work in rigorous clinical studies. It's Holism, reproducibility and ease of practice and application depends upon unique basic principles which comprises of profound but well-systematized philosophical principles that provide valuable hypotheses of holistic preventions and treatment. It also includes the mandatories of testing these hypotheses by rigorous scientific experimentation and observation.

The remarkable Holism of Persian doctrine of Medicine arises from giving primacy to the Temperament of man and drug, which unlike the molecular level, is simple and can be known as a whole. Its ease of practice arises from the fact that it uses only a few parameters i.e. the primary qualities of Hot: Cold & Dry: Wet to describe the temperament of both man and drug. Its precision and reproducibility arises from the principle of clinical testing of the drugs hypothesized by Temperament, before accepting them. This clinical testing also reveals effects which cannot be deduced from the temperament or basic qualities of the drug.

The basic principles comprise of:

- The Seven Natural Factors, essential factors for the constitution of human body
- The basics of Pathology
- The Principles of Diagnosis
- The Principles of Treatment

The Natural Factors

Persian doctrine of Medicine describes man to be made up of the following seven factors:

a) Elements: What man and the Universe, both biological and non-biological, including drugs are made up of.

b) Humors: The form taken up by elements in living things. Their balance is health while imbalance is disease.

c) Temperament: It is the general quality of man, drug etc. due to the quality of dominant elements. It is used as the qualitative yardstick for measuring health and deviation from it, and for identifying the drugs that can restore the balance. It is the basis of constitutional medicine.

d) Organs: The physical body.

e) Pneuma: The subtle substance having vitality, and acting as carrier of physiological powers.

f) Faculties: The physiological powers responsible for Corresponding basic functions of the organism i.e. life, nutrition, sensation, movement and reproduction.

g) Functions: Functions of various organs.

Elements: Basic elements in Persian Medicine are simple indivisible matters which provide the primary components for the human body and others. They cannot be further resolved into simpler entities. The various substances (compounds) in nature depend for their existence on their chemical compositions. Everything in the Universe is composed of four basic elements in varying amount and proportion. Each element has two sets of basic qualities: Hot or Cold and Dry or Wet. The four elements are Fire, Air, Water and Earth. Their basic qualities are:

Fire: Hot & Dry

Air : Hot & Wet

Water: Cold & Wet

Earth: Cold & Dry

All things including man and drug are made up of these four basic elements combined in different amount and proportion. Each thing is characterized by a new quality arising from the proportion and interaction of its constituent elements. These individual qualities can be broadly classified into four basic groups: Hot & Dry, Hot & Wet, Cold & Wet and Cold & Dry.

The Humors are the liquid fundamental substance of living things, made up by the mixing and organic transformation of elements and thereby obtaining the ability to support biological processes i.e. life, nutrition & growth, sensation & movement and reproduction. The Humors are four in number and characterized by the dominant basic Qualities:

The Humors are formed within various organs, primarily in liver and run together in the blood vessels. They have both Subtle and Gross components. Subtle components mix to form Pneuma while Gross components give rise to the physical organs and body. Although each Humor is made up by the mixing of Four Elements, but corresponds to a particular element on the basis of the dominant quality. Every individual has a unique humoral composition which represents his specific temperament.

However, these Temperaments show variations within a range depending on age, sex, race, geographical distribution, environment etc. The gross deviation from this unique balance due to any cause is disease. The diseases can be classified according to the abnormally dominant Humor. The collection of imbalance by applying drugs and other factors having the opposite temperament results in cure.

Temperament

Human Beings are classifiable into four types which characterizes their entire being: body, mind and pneuma. Each type is associated with a dominant Humor and named accordingly as:

Sanguine: Hot & Wet

Choleric: Hot & Dry

Phlegmatic: Cold & Wet

Melancholic: Cold & Dry

However, the temperament can also be described in terms of the basic qualities, as shown in the second column. A person's well-being and proper treatment, in case of falling ill, depends upon eating, living and medicating in light of his/her temperament.

Drugs, diet, geographical regions, seasons, professional environment and even the individual organs and body parts of man etc. all are characterized by respective temperaments. So, it is possible to make the necessary correlations between the temperament of man and the temperament of these factors. However, their temperament is expressed in terms of the basic qualities, whereas, man's temperament is expressed in terms of Humors, which, however, is easily translatable into basic qualities.

The temperament of man can be diagnosed by ten categories of bodily and mental parameters, e.g. complexion, texture, built, hair, psychic reactions etc. The pathological change of temperament, in whole man or in particular body parts and organs, can also be diagnosed by changes in these parameters.

Organs

The physical body is made up of Organs/Tissues. They are of two types: Simple and Compound. The simple organs are tissues like fat, bone etc. while compound organs are poly-tissue structures like heart, brain, liver etc.

Pneumas

The pneuma is subtle, physical substance made from the subtle components of the Humors. It possesses vitality and provides life to the organism. It also acts as the seat and carrier of the physiological powers or faculties which are responsible for producing the corresponding physiological processes, e.g. nutrition & growth, sensation & movement etc.

Man possesses three pneumas, each generated in a vital organ:

Vital pneuma: Heart

Psychic Pneuma: Brain

Natural Pneuma: Liver

Since, the faculties subsist in the pneuma, derangements of the temperament of the pneuma can vitiate the functions of the faculties and the restoration of the temperament of pneuma by drugs of opposite temperament will restore the function. Mind corresponds to the psychic faculty which subsists in psychic pneuma. So, Persian doctrine of Medicine treats mental diseases mainly by using drugs to rebalance the temperament of the psychic pneuma. Thus, Persian doctrine of Medicine is very successful in curing psychiatric diseases by treating the mind as a substance.

Faculties

These are the physiological powers that give rise to corresponding physiological functions. The faculties are non-substantial powers that can exist in the organism only by subsisting in the corresponding pneuma. The primary faculties, their carrier pneuma and their functions are as follows:

The faculties get drawn and attached to the corresponding pneuma as soon as the pneuma attains their proper temperament.

Functions: They are the physiological functions and processes undergoing in organs and tissues due to the operation of faculties or physiological powers.

Classical Persian Medicine research methodology

Persian doctrine of Medicine not only described basic principles, extensive clinical descriptions of diseases and thousands of medicaments and formulations but it also laid down, hundreds of years ago, a precise research methodology: Treatment of a disease should be inferred by determining the temperament of a disease and the temperament of the drug to be used in particular disease. The temperament of the drug must be compatible with the temperament of the patient on the principles of Heterotherapy and these conclusions should be tested by rigorous scientific testing. It also had the principle that some drug effects cannot be inferred by any general theory and can be discovered only by empirical study.

Thus, it is a medicine that along with having a deep and easy to apply philosophical vision, provided importance and space to empirical scientific testing. Due to effective philosophical principles, it succeeded in maintaining its philosophy-based holism.

Disease process

The Persian doctrine of Medicine defines health and disease state. In great majority of illnesses, the disease is basically an imbalance in the normal temperament and also comprises of disorganization and discontinuity of structure. However, these three basic pathologies may exist independently too.

States of the body

According to Persian doctrine of Medicine states of the body are grouped under two heads:

Health in which all the functions of the body are in the range normal for a particular individual.

Disease is the opposite of Health in which one or more functions or forms of the bodily organs are at fault.

Disease

Disease amounts to a pathological condition of the body which is provoked by a cause. They are of two types:

Single disease

Complex disease

A single disease may manifest itself in any of the following three forms:

Dyscrasia: The temperament wherein the qualities and quantities of all the participating elements in a compound are not in accordance with what the compound is made for.

Structural diseases: Abnormality of Structure

Diseases of dissolution of Unity

Complex disease is a combination of two or more single diseases.

Cause

Cause corresponds with the etiology. It can be defined as a specific factor which either maintain the state of the body or changes it from health to sickness or from sickness to health. Causes of diseases can be divided into two types: External causes and internal causes. External causes are those which affect the body from outside such as excessive hot or cold climate, a polluted atmosphere, injury etc. Internal causes are those which appear and affect the body internally such as formation of stones inside the kidney or bladder.

Secondary Abnormality

Secondary abnormality arises from the basic pathology. In diarrhea, for example, dehydration is a major secondary abnormality.

The basic pathology and the secondary pathology can be diagnosed by the particular signs and symptoms.

Principles of diagnosis and treatment

In accordance with its holistic vision of man and disease, Persian doctrine of Medicine uses macroscopic parameters rather than microscopic or biochemical parameters for diagnosis. Since, its holism also takes into account the subtle level of man. Therefore, Persian doctrine of Medicine also uses subjective parameters, such as dreams. However, its diagnostic system is very sophisticated and accurate and succeeds in diagnosing diseases in a reproducible manner. Secondly, being macroscopic, it is highly economical and independent of technological paraphernalia. It also has the conceptual framework to use modern medical diagnostic means in some cases where they are useful at a secondary level. For instance, since it considers discontinuity in structure as a basic pathology, it has no hesitation in using endoscopy to see extent of gut ulceration after diagnosing the basic pathology by its macroscopic method.

The unique holistic diagnostics of Persian doctrine of Medicine comprises of History, Physical Examination. Pulse Examination and Inspection of Excreta.

History taking and physical examination

It is undertaken according to general parameters and the specific parameters required by the particular problem of the patient, guided mainly by the 'Ten Fundamental Categories'.

Pulse

The pulse is fundamentally observed in the light of ten parameters. Apart from these, some other types of compound pulses have also been described in Persian doctrine of medicine. Further, the specific type of pulse in each disease is also described, mainly in the light of the general parameters.

Iranian physicians judge the nature of the functional disturbance of the human system empirically by examining the pulse of a patient. This judgment is based on the experience of the individual physician.

Pulse is examined by ten features; size, strength, speed, consistency (elasticity), fullness, temperature, rate, frequency (constancy), regularity and rhythm.

Persian Medicine scholars have described pulse under several headings such as normal pulse, factors governing the pulse, effects of patient factors such as sex, age, temperament and season, region and country, food and drink, sleep and wakefulness, exercise, bath, pregnancy, pain, swelling, emotions and of factors inimical to the body.

Physical Examination of Urine

Physical examination of urine helps a lot in the diagnosis, not only of uro-genital diseases but other systemic disorders. For this following aspects are taken into account:

Quantity, color, odor, consistency, foam or froth, clearness and turbidity, sediment

Physical Examination of Stool

The physical examination of stool also helps in the diagnosis of various diseases. Color, quantity, consistency and the presence of foreign bodies are observed during physical examination

Management of diseases in Persian Medicine

In Persian doctrine of medicine, the management of diseases depends upon the pathology involved in the disease process. These principles are as under:

Removal of the causative factor: the causative factors in the pathology of the disease process are determined and removed for the proper management of the disease.

Normalization of the dys-temperament: the disease in which, the temperament of a person is altered without affecting the quality and quantity of humors, only correction of simple morbid temperament is required. This is achieved simply by modifying the lifestyle of the patient in view of essential and non-essential factors.

Evacuation of morbid material: if the temperament is changed due to increase in the quantity and volume of certain humors and that morbid material in the body gets accumulated, it is evacuated by various therapies through different routes for the cure of the disease e.g. cupping, venesection, leeching, concoctive purgative therapy, expectoration, diuresis, diaphoresis etc.

Hetero-therapy: this is the main principle of treatment in Persian doctrine of medicine, in which the drug having opposite temperament to the disease is administered for the correction of morbid temperament and cure of illness.

Surgical and Para-surgical procedures: in Persian doctrine of medicine, diseases of the structure and breach of continuity are treated by using suitable operative and Para-operative techniques as applied for the treatment by the Persian Medicine scholars.

Psychiatric Treatment: the Persian doctrine of medicine treats psychiatric diseases by using drugs, modifying mind-related processes like sleep and psychotherapy. it is able to use drugs by its discovery of the 'substance of mind' i.e. psychic pneuma while its appreciation of the medical importance of processes, physical conditions etc., which it organizes as 'six essential factors', helps it to closely relate sleep etc. to the improvement of psychiatric and psycho-somatic diseases. It also makes use of psychotherapy by manipulative techniques of mind by verbal means. but its main reliance is on drug treatment as it has discovered the subtle substance of mind and its relation with drugs due to their common temperament.

Spiritual Treatment: the Persian doctrine of medicine recognizes the role of spiritual health and treatment by discovering that the spirit is joined to the pneuma and through them, to the body, and is the supreme regulator of man. However, they restrict itself only to the pneuma and body, and leaves spiritual treatment to religious and spiritual counseling by spiritual experts. Although, it does not oblige the physician to be a spiritual authority but culturally most physicians are also spiritually advanced and provide religious and spiritual counseling which has a powerful role in healthcare by facilitating a healthy lifestyle and by distressing the patient.

Three primary sources of drugs: in Persian doctrine of medicine, drugs obtained only from herbal, animal and mineral sources are used for medication. Somtimes, these drugs are used singly, and Somtimes in the form of a compound of various drugs. They may be subjected to physico-chemical processing but without breaking up their natural character. Thus, Persian doctrine of medicine uses only natural substances in treatment.

Preventive healthcare

Persian Medicine has the methods of understanding and maintaining health in a positive and individualized manner, with different guidelines for different temperaments, genders, age-groups, geographical regions, seasons, occupations etc.

Maintenance of health is followed by methods for preventing disease. it should be noted that it describes not only prevention of disease but promotion of what it calls maintenance of health as a separate discipline, which should be used even before prevention of disease. This is because, being holistic, it possesses a positive concept and description of health. Though, understandably quite elaborate, the section on treatment of diseases comes only after preventive guidelines.

Like treatment of disease, maintenance of health is also based upon both deeply profound principles, and rigorous testing and experimentation. As in treatment of disease, so in promotion of health and prevention of disease, the most basic principle is temperament. in disease, treatment is done by using non-drug and drug factors of opposite temperament, while for maintenance of health, mostly non-drug factors of the same temperament are used .

Six essential factors

The observational and philosophic genius of Persian Medicine scientists found one of its best expressions in the six essential factors, whose appropriate deployment in the life of a person, determined by their temperament, and ensures health. in fact, Iranian scientific describes all the factors affecting health and disease, of whom those affecting all human beings perpetually are called essential while, the rest are called non-essential.

The essential factors cover a very wide range, and their creatively thought out applications or rectifications are even more numerous. For instance, pure and profuse air is essential for health. These six essential factors are remarkable in providing such six categories that can include a very large number of factors, which may outwardly be quite distant to each other. It should be noted that the 'six essential factors' are used not only for maintaining health and preventing diseases, but also for treating diseases.

These six essential principles are as: air, foods and drinks, movement and rest, mental movement and repose, sleep and wakefulness, evacuation and retention

Air

Air is the most crucial factor for life. It helps in the production and maintenance of pneuma which is the source of vitality. From the perspective of Persian Medicine clear air is the air without any chemical contaminants. Persian doctrine of medicine uses air in prevention and treatment chiefly by taking into account the seasonal variations in air. For instance, in summer, air becomes hotter so cold food and moderate movement and exercise should be adopted to remain health.

Foods and drinks

Food is second only to air in maintaining life and health by replacing the body's used-up and broken-down components. Keeping in view the importance of food, Persian doctrine of medicine makes extensive use of diet both for promotion of health and treatment of disease. It has been very successful in identifying the appropriate food by using the principle of temperament. a healthy man should use mainly the food of the temperament similar to his own temperament. However, if he is threatened with a pathological shift in his temperament, he should use food of the opposite temperament. Many diseases are caused by lack of attention to appropriate food and life style of people. It's necessary for human being, to pay attention to choose what he/she eats to balance temperament.

Movement and Rest

The Persian doctrine of medicine gives great importance to both appropriate movement and rest for maintaining health and for curing disease. Movement is necessary for evacuating waste products, and rest is needed for retaining nutrients till the completion of digestion. They offer a wide concept of exercise of all organs. It classifies movement into two types: high frequency and intensity with short duration, which increases heat; and low frequency and intensity with long duration, which increases metabolism. It recommends moderate exercise, which produces moderate sweating, but discourages intense exercise, which produces profuse sweating.

Mental movement and repose

Persian Medicine scientists fully recognize the role of psychic states in maintaining health and treating disease. They describe mental states basically in terms of the mental movement and repose. Movement increases heat while repose increases cold, so excessive movement or repose of pneuma causes hot and cold pathologies.

Thus, these pathologies can be managed both by altering the mental states and by administering cold or hot drugs. This is the basis of the unique and successful psycho- pharmacological management of psychiatric and psychosomatic diseases in Persian Medicine.

In addition to considering the pneuma as basic to mental states, Persian Medicine considers the heart and the brain to be especially relevant, as heart is the seat of pneuma and the soul, while, brain is the seat of psychic faculties. So mental states - described by Persian Medicine in terms of psychic movement and repose - specially affect heart and brain function. it must also be appreciated that, since Persian Medicine considers heart function to be basically the maintenance of vitality (energy and immunity), therefore, it describes close correlation of mental states with immunity

Sleep and Wakefulness

Sleep is necessary for preserving pneuma and vitality and providing replacement of wear and tear, while wakefulness is necessary for voluntary functions. Since, they resemble repose and movement, respectively, excess of sleep increases coldness and wetness, while excess of wakefulness increases hotness and dryness. Therefore, moderation should be exercised with regard to them. Just as wakefulness helps voluntary functions, particularly intellectual functions, sleep helps digestion. So the digestion of hot food is more dependent on sleep.

Evacuation and Retention

Evacuation is needed for removal of waste products which may cause obstructions or embolism and toxicity. Retention of nutrients etc. is needed not only for full digestion and metabolism but also to maintain reserves of nutrients and essential substances. Evacuation takes place by defecation, micturition, coitus, sweating etc. Persian doctrine of medicine puts great emphasis on proper evacuation and prescribes mild laxatives like for managing mild constipation. it also encourages all those activities in moderation that lead to evacuation, e.g. coitus and bath etc. .

Therapeutic approaches

Treatment is adopted when prevention fails and disease occurs. It is mainly based upon hetero-therapy. Disease, which amounts to the emergence of an abnormal temperament, is treated by applying drugs and non-drug factors with opposite temperament.

Thus, Persian doctrine of medicine describes following modes of treatment:

•Regimental therapy

•Dietotherapy

•Pharmacotherapy

•Manipulative techniques

Regimental therapy

Regimental therapy is one of the most popular methods of treatment, practiced by Iranian physicians since antiquity. Literally, *'tadbir'* is an Arabic word meaning 'regimen' or 'systematic plan' whereas 'elaj' means 'therapy' or 'treatment'. Thus, 'elaj by tadbir' means treatment through regimen, by which care of the sick person is taken and the general health is maintained. In this way, Regimental therapy comprises mostly non-medicinal procedures by which the lifestyles for preservation of health and treatment of disease are modulated. Iranian physicians, e.g. Rhazes and Avicenna have described various regimens for the management of diseases, either independently or in combination with other therapies. These include changes in diet, physical exercise, lifestyle modification and measures to eliminate the morbid Humors from the body or divert them by Cupping, Massage, Leeching, Venesection, Purgation, Emesis, Diuresis, Enema, Diaphoresis, Expectoration, Counter Irritation, Sitz Bath etc. Some other regimens are also used for elimination/diversion of morbid material or resolution of the inflammation, e.g. bath, Irrigation, Fomentation etc.

Cupping

Cupping is a technique in which a cup is applied over the surface of skin by creating vacuum and it is known as dry cupping Somtimes, scarification is done at the location of cupping to draw blood from the body part to relieve internal congestion, and this process is known as wet cupping.

The objectives of Cupping are as follows:

- To eliminate/divert the morbid material
- To enhance the blood supply and correct cold temperament or to rectify the temperament of a particular organ
- To achieve antispasmodic and detoxifying effect
- To evacuate waste products through skin

Leeching

Leeching is a method of elimination of morbid matter from the body. In this procedure, Leeches are applied on the affected part to suck the blood from deeper tissues. During this process, the leeches also infuse their saliva into the blood, which is a complex mixture of different biologically and pharmacologically active substances. Recently, various studies have been conducted to validate these methods in various diseases, e.g. Arthritis, Hypertension, Skin disorders etc.

Venesection

Venesection is a method of absolute elimination, used to remove the excess of Humors or to get rid of morbid matter from the body. In this procedure, an incision is given to the superficial veins and blood is allowed to flow. The objectives of the procedure are as follows:

- To remove excess of Humors
- To prevent toxicity and accumulation of waste material in blood
- To excrete the waste material from various part of body
- To stimulation metabolic processes
- To correct the altered temperament

Bath

Bath is a place used for bathing, consisting of several rooms with one room leading to the other with specific provisions and conditions customized according to the disease to be treated. The objectives of Bath are as follows:

- To reduce viscosity of the Humors
- To improve health in the debilitated individuals
- To increase innate heat of the body

• To improve metabolism

• To evacuate waste products through skin

• To treat the paralysis and muscular wasting

• To strengthen the body

• To cure obesity

Massage

Massage is a manipulative technique of superficial and deeper layers of muscle and connective tissues using various techniques, to enhance body functions, healing process, and promote relaxation and well-being. Various types of Massage have been recommended in Persian Medicine for the management of various disorders. The objectives of Massage are as follows:

• To increase weight

• To relieve psychosomatic disorders

• To relieve backache, headache, and muscular pain

Physical exercise

Physical exercise is any voluntary movement of body or its part that enhances or maintains physical fitness and overall health. It plays an important role not only in maintaining good health and prevention of diseases but also in curing certain ailments. The objectives of physical exercise are as follows:

• To improve metabolism

• To tone up the organs/systems

• To maintain or improve flexibility, co-ordination and balance of the musculoskeletal system

- To strengthen the body as a whole

- To relieve anxiety, insomnia and depression

- To remove waste products from the body

Diuresis

Diuresis is a process in which formation and excretion of urine is increased for the management of bodily ailments. It is one of the important processes adopted for evacuation of morbid matter from the body through urine. Diuresis can be induced by adopting specific methods like exposure to cold, drinking of cold water and intake of plenty of fluids. It can also be induced with the help of certain drugs that have been mentioned in classical Persian Medicine literature under the heading of Diuretics. The objectives of Diuresis are as follows:

- To excrete waste products and excess of Humors through urine

- To purify blood and evacuate morbid Humors

- To manage diseases of heart, kidney and liver

Purgation

Purgation is a method of elimination of waste and morbid matter from the body through rectum. During this process, the frequency of stool is increased by decreasing the absorption of water in the intestines, by increasing the peristaltic movement or both.

Emesis

Emesis is the evacuation of gastric contents through mouth. The main purpose of emesis is to eliminate toxic/morbid material from the upper gastro-intestinal tract. The objectives of emesis are as follows:

- To manage gastro-intestinal diseases

• To manage diseases like Headache, Migraine, Melancholia etc.

Diaphoresis

Diaphoresis is a process of induced sweating. It is instrumental in liquefying the sticky and adherent Humors lodged in the peripheral tissues. The objectives of diaphoresis are as follows:

• To excrete the waste matter from the skin

• To reduce the excessive heat

• To divert the morbid material from kidney to the skin

• To purify blood

• To improve dermal nutrition and enhance body texture

Cauterization

Cauterization is an effective method of treating several conditions e.g. destructive lesions, removal of putrefactive matter, stoppage of bleeding etc. Iranian physicians have been using this method over the centuries. The instrument used for cauterization is called as cautery preferably made up of gold.

Concoctive and Purgative Therapy

It is the main method of treatment for the chronic diseases in Persian doctrine of Medicine. It is actually meant for evacuation or elimination of morbid Humors from the body. Morbid Humors are mainly responsible for aggravating the disease process if they remain stagnant in the body. Abnormal Humors are evacuated from the body by a method known as elimination. Somtimes the matter is too thick or too thin to be eliminated properly Therefore, some drugs are used that change the consistency of the morbid Humor and make it suitable for elimination. Such drugs are known as concoctive. For each Humor, specific concoctive drugs are used to make the morbid Humor able to be evacuated. For example, in phlegmatic diseases Lavandula stoechas

(Ustukhudus) is used as a concoctive. Once the features of concoction are established in the respective Humor, it is followed by purgation.

Psychiatric Treatment

Persian doctrine of Medicine has emphasized the importance of psychiatric and psychological factors including spiritual values in the management of various diseases. The therapy compliments conventional medicine by treating the whole person - mind, body and spirit. This therapy has been described under the heading of Psychiatric Treatment. The benefits of the therapy may be felt on physical and emotional level. Iranian physicians have described the psychiatric treatment for various psychotic and psychosomatic disorders such as Anxiety neurosis. However, Persian doctrine of Medicine uses drugs very effectively in Psychiatric Diseases. This is so because the Persian Medicine counterpart of Mind is Psychic Pneuma which is made up of subtle matter and possesses Temperament. Therefore, the psychiatric diseases are characterized by various pathological Temperaments and can be easily treated by drugs of opposite Temperament.

Dietotherapy

Persian doctrine of Medicine lays great stress on treating certain ailments by administration of specific diets or by regulating the quality and quantity of food. In addition to nutritional properties, various foods have pharmacological actions too. For example, many foods are laxative, diuretic and diaphoretic.

The weakness of certain organs is corrected by administering the same organ of an animal by way of food: for instance, disorders and weakness of liver are treated by including the goat liver in the patient's diet. Likewise, heart, kidney and brain are recommended in the respective organ's treatment.

Pharmacotherapy

According to Persian doctrine of Medicine, the choice of drugs for treatment is governed by three laws:

(i) Quality of drug in terms of Temperament,

(ii) Quantity of drug in terms of its weight and potency and

(iii) Time of administration

The selection of drug depends on the nature and type of the disease. The proper drug is that which its pathological Temperament is contrary to the nature and qualitative pattern of the disease i.e. The weight and potency of the drug is determined by the nature of the organ; severity of the disease: and other related factors such as sex, age, weight, habit and habitat, season, built, previous treatment, and stage of the disease.

The Persian doctrine of Medicine states that the drugs have their own particular temperament due to their specific constituents. Concoctive drugs are used to prepare the morbid matter for excretion, whereas Purgative drugs are used to remove morbid matter through intestine.

Persian Medicine drugs are used in different forms e.g. Powder, decoction, infusion, tablet, semisolid preparations. In Heterotherapy, drugs having qualities and temperament opposite to those present in the diseases should be administered.

Surgery

Surgery has always been a part of treatment in Persian doctrine of Medicine since ancient times.

Drugs

The Persian doctrine of Medicine describes the general character of a drug in terms of its Temperament. By correlating it with the temperament of the disease it is able to eradicate the disease as a whole i.e. achieve holistic treatment. Secondly, as the temperament of the drug indicates its pharmacological actions, e.g. a Hot & Dry Drug may be Lithotryptic (breaking of renal stone), and the temperament can be determined by physical properties such as taste etc. and by the effect on temperaments in human beings. So, it is possible to propose or hypothesize the actions of a drug by the simple means of determining its temperament. However, Persian doctrine of Medicine enjoins that the pharmacological action thus hypothesized on the basis of temperament should be clinically tested before being recommended as treatment. In addition to Temperament, a second basis of Pharmacological Actions is also described i.e. the Essence.

Secondly, the Persian doctrine of Medicine uses only natural products as drugs. This is one of the basic reasons of its safety. However, it discovered and used advanced chemical processing e.g. distillation, sublimation etc. for drug formulation which increase their selectivity, efficacy, and palatability. But, care is taken not to disturb the basic natural character of drugs. Thus, Persian doctrine of Medicine is unique in achieving a golden balance between naturality and physico-chemical processing, and obtains the benefits and advantages of both.

Iran has a rich flora, which are used as drugs in Persian doctrine of Medicine. In spite of great advances made in modem medicine during the last few decades, plants still have an important role in healthcare. It is estimated that about 25 percent of all the allopathic drugs are directly or indirectly derived from the plants. In some particular cases, such as antitumor and antimicrobial drugs, about 60 percent of the medicines currently available in the market are from natural products. This underscores the efficacy of natural products. However, Persian doctrine of Medicine uses the natural products as a whole rather than their active ingredients. So, Persian Medicine treatment is safe, efficacious, and easily available: and hence, widely acceptable.

In Persian doctrine of Medicine, there is a unique concept of Food Medicine and Medicinal Food. Substances used primarily for their medicinal properties but also having nutritional value are called Food Medicine e.g. Almond. Therefore, they not only treat a disease but also nourish the patient. The substances which are used primarily as food but also have some medicinal properties are known as Medicinal Food e.g. Egg. They have the advantage of being very safe.

Drug Source

Only natural substances are used as drugs. Although Persian doctrine of Medicine made great advancements in the chemical processing of drugs i.e. distillation, sublimation etc. it did not disturb the basic natural character of drugs, which is one of the fundamental reasons for the safety of Persian Medicine Drugs. Thus, products from all the three natural sources i.e. plants, minerals and animals are used as drugs.

Based on their origin, the Persian Medicine drugs are classified into three categories:

Drugs of plant origin: Roots, stems, bark, leaves, flower, seed, fruit, gum, resin, extract etc.

Drugs of mineral origin: Different metals: metal ores and non-metals in the natural form.

Drugs of animal origin: Animal glands, tissues and certain animal poisons.

Principles of drug action

Persian Medicine drugs act either by their Temperament or by their Essence. The Temperament of a drug can be determined by its basic qualities viz. hot, cold, dry or wet, which then indicate certain pharmacological actions, which have to be confirmed by clinical testing.

Temperament of Drugs

Like all entities of the Universe, Drugs are also constituted by the mixing of Elements. Therefore, their basic character is indicated by the resulting qualitative Temperament, e.g. hot drugs, Cold drugs etc. When it is said that a drug is hot or cold, it does not mean that it is intrinsically very hot or cold, or that it is hotter or colder than the human body. Rather, it indicates that such a drug produces a greater degree of heat or cold in the body than what was originally present. Further, the same drug may be less hot for one person than for the other. This is one of the reasons why different drugs are prescribed for the same disease in different persons.

Categories of Drugs

Pharmacological Actions arise from the Qualities of the Drug indicated by its Temperament. Therefore, potency of a drug is described by grading the Temperament into four degrees:

First degree drugs: First degree drugs do produce pharmacological effects but their effects, in terms of Qualities i.e. hot or cold, are not perceptible.

Second degree drugs: The effect of these drugs, in terms of qualities, are perceptible, but not to the extent of altering the normal functioning of the body.

Third degree drugs: The effects of these drugs, in terms of qualities, are strong and alter the normal functioning of body significantly, but not to the extent of causing harm.

Fourth degree drugs: The effects of these drugs are excessively strong and toxic to the extent of being fatal. However, these drugs can be used safely after undergoing specific process.

Pharmaceutics

The Persian doctrine of Medicine prescribes elaborate formulation or pharmaceutical processing of drugs for achieving stability, palatability, absorption and assimilability, and for enhancing efficacy and safety. These objectives are obtained not only by developing various dosage forms on rational and experimental bases but also by devising many processing techniques. This pharmaceutical processing is applied to both Single (Single ingredient) Preparations and Compound (Multiple

Ingredient) Preparations, majority being of the later type. It also has a unique specialty of adding Collective Drugs to counter the toxicity of the main drug.

The Persian Medicine Drugs are being manufactured mostly in the classical form. Modern instruments are used in preparation of drugs. Somtimes, minor alterations are made in the dosage forms, and due care is taken not to depart from the essence. The Persian Medicine Drug Industry is preparing and marketing two types of drugs: (i) Classical Persian Medicine formulations (ii) Patent and Proprietary products. Good Manufacturing Practices are followed in order to ensure quality control of these drugs.

Dosage Forms

The dosage forms have been developed to achieve all the basic objectives of pharmaceutical processing i.e. palatability, assimilability, stability and the enhancement of safety and efficacy. In Persian doctrine of Medicine, drugs are used mainly in four forms viz. solid, semi-solid, and liquid and vapors. Solid dosage forms are Pill, Tablet, and Powder etc. Semi-solid dosage forms are of various types. Liquid dosage forms are decoction, infusion, distillate, syrup, drops etc. Vapor dosage forms are fumigation and steam inhalation, perfumes, etc. In addition to the oral drugs Persian Medicine physicians also administer the drugs through enema, Sitz bath, pessary, suppository, liniment etc.

Besides, "calyx means Koshteh" are used for various ailments. "Koshteh" are fine powdered form of medicinal preparations obtained by the calcination of metal, mineral and animal origin drugs along with potentiating and corrective herbs which convert them into organic forms that become biologically assailable. The word "Koshteh" is derived from "koshtan" - a Persian word meaning "to kill" that denotes all the above changes. It should be noted that the inclusion of herbs prescribed by Persian doctrine of Medicine produces additional qualities.

Specific processing of drugs

Persian Medicine scholars were aware that the drugs of the fourth degree - drawn from plants, minerals (metals) and animals, are toxic and harmful to the body. However, if they properly processed become safe enough for therapeutic use. Many techniques are used for the processing of drugs. Comparative Pharmacological studies of the natural and processed forms of toxic drugs like Arsenic, Aconitum lapillus etc. have revealed that the processed forms practically lose their toxicity when compared with the unprocessed, natural form.

The objectives of Processing in Persian doctrine of Medicine are not limited to detoxification but also include efficacy enhancement and pharmacokinetic optimization i.e. achievement of desirable rate of absorption, delivery to target tissue etc. A very large number of innovative processing techniques have been developed in Persian doctrine of Medicine. Some of the important techniques are as follows:

Burning

This process is undertaken to evaporate the moisture content and to make the drug completely dry as indicated in respective formula. Drugs are burnt to the charring stage but not reduced to ash.

Bathing

In this process the drugs are ground to fine powder. Thereafter, sufficient quantity of water is added, stirred and allowed to settle down. The coarse particles will settle down at the bottom. The finer particles of the stone still suspended in the water will come out when decanted. The decanted water is left undisturbed so that the finest particles are settled down at the bottom, water is removed, and the particles when dried are finely powdered.

Roasting

In this process the drugs are roasted to evaporate the moisture for their easy powdering, and to enhance their absorption.

Frying

In this process the drugs are fried in a suitable oil to purify them and reduce the toxicity.

Tashvieh

In this process the drugs are wrapped into mud or wheat dough, kept in hot ash for a specified period, removed, unwrapped and squeezed to collect their juices for medicinal use.

Purification

In this process solution of drug is slowly passed through a filtering medium. Some of the plant-animal- and mineral origin drugs are naturally toxic in their properties and actions. Therefore, these drugs are detoxified or purified before adding in the formulation, in order to reduce their toxicity and enhance therapeutic action.

Calyx

For preparation of "calyx", the drugs are ground and converted into tablet, put into the earthen pot, and sealed by layers of cloth and clay. These are subjected to calcination by placing them in a pit between layers of cow dung cakes. The latter are then ignited. The intensity of heat is adjusted by specified number of cow dung cakes and dimensions of the pit. After calcination, the pit is allowed to cool completely. The earthen plates are taken out and the contents collected. Persian Medicine scholars prepared "calyx" for deep penetration, rapid action, long shelf life and better efficacy of the drug.

Corrective Drugs

The scholars of the Persian doctrine of Medicine were aware of various possible adverse effects of some of the drugs. Therefore, while describing the characteristics of drugs they mentioned their possible adverse effects, along with their Corrective Drugs.

BIBLIOGRAPHY

1. Avicenna. The Canon of Medicine. Beirut, Lebanon. Institute of scientific Publication; 2003.
2. Organization. WH. The promotion and development of medicine: report of a WHO meeting.: World Health Organ Tech Rep Ser; 1978. p. 1-41.
3. Aghili Khorasani MH. Research institute for islamic and complementary medicine. Tehran, Iran: Kholasat-ol-hekmat; 2006.
4. Naseri M, Namavar H. Maintaining Health in the view point of "TIM". Tehran, Iran: Institute for "Traditional Iranian Medicine" Publication; 2014.
5. Hysen P. timeline of graeco-arabic medicine. An introduction to graeco-arabic medicine: Graeco-arabic medicine society inc; 2000.
6. Ebrahimnejad H. Religion and Medicine in Iran," History of Science. 2002; 60:91-112.
7. Tan SY. Hippocrates: father of medicine.
8. Jackson WA. A short guide to humoral medicine. Trends in pharmacological sciences. 2001 Sep 1; 22(9):487.
9. Pormann PE, Savage-Smith E, Hehmeyer I. Medieval Islamic Medicine. Edinburgh: Edinburgh University Press; 2007 Jan.
10. Khan MS. Islamic medicine. Routledge; 2013 Oct 16.
11. Tibi S. Al-Razi and Islamic medicine in the 9th Century. Journal of the Royal Society of Medicine. 2006 Apr 1; 99(4):206-7.
12. Hamarneh S. Medical education and practice in medieval Islam.
13. Cyril E. A Medical History of Persia and the Eastern Caliphate. Published by: The Syndics of the Cambridge University Press, Printed in Great Britain at the University Press, Cambridge. 1951:9.
14. Osler W. Evolution of modern medicine. DevCom; 1921.
15. Shah MH, editor. The general principles of Avicenna's Canon of Medicine. Naveed Clinic; 1966.
16. A translation of the Books I-II was made by Laleh Bakhtiar (Bakhtiar, 1999).

17. Abu-Asab M, Amri H, Micozzi MS. Avicenna's medicine: a new translation of the 11th-century canon with practical applications for integrative health care. Simon and Schuster; 2013 Jul 4.
18. Zillur Rahman, H.S. (1986). Qanoon lbn Sina Aur Uskey Shareheen wa Mutarjemeen. Publication Division, Aligarh Muslim University, Aligarh 1986; 2nd ed., 2012. Translated by Zakaria Virk: Commentators and Translations of Ibn Sina's Canon of Medicine, 2012.
19. Sigerist HE. A history of medicine: Early Greek, Hindu, and Persian medicine. New York: Oxford University Press; 1987.
20. Lindlahr H. Philosophy of natural therapeutics. Lindlahr Publishing Co. 1922.
21. Ebne Nafis A. Almojaz fi teb.: Ghahereh Publication; 2001.
22. Hakim GMC. The healer's handbook: A classic guide to the medicine of avicenna paperback. 1988.
23. Mones AA, Hakima A, Marc S. Micozzi ,avicenna's medicine: A new translation of the 11th-century canon with practical applications for integrative health care. 2013.
24. Aghili Khorasani MH. Research institute for islamic and complementary medicine. Tehran, Iran: Kholasat-ol-hekmat; 2006.
25. Jorjani E. Researchinstitute for islamic and complementary medicine. Tehran, Iran: Zakhireh Kharazmshahi; 2002.
26. Ahvazi A. Kamelo senae tebieh.: Jalaladin Publication; 2008.
27. Avicenna. Canon of medicine (translated into English by Hameed HA. S. Waris Nawab, Senior Press Superintendent). Jamia Hamdard Printing Press; 1998.
28. Gilani MK. Hefzo sehe naseri.: Almei Publication; 2008.
29. Arzani MA. Teb e Akbari. Tehran, Iran: Research institute for islamic and complementary medicine; 2008.
30. Kermani NE. Share asbab va alamat.: Jalaladin Publication; 2008.
31. Jorjani EBH. Khofi Alaee.: Etelaat Publication; 1990.
32. Razi Z. Alhavi fi Teb. Beyroot: Dar Ehia alteras alarabi; 2001.
33. Razi MBZ. Mansori fi teb. Tehran, Iran: Tehran university of medical science, institute for islamic and complementary medicine; 2008.
34. Kermani MKBE. Daghaegh ol Alaj. Saadat Publication; 1983.

35. Mosaddegh M, Naghibi F. Iran's medicine, past and present, medicine and materia medica. Tehran, Iran: TMRC; 2002.
36. Jorjani SE. Aghrazo tebieh va mabaheso alaeeieh.: Tehran university of medical science publication; 2003.

Made in United States
Orlando, FL
04 November 2026

90200103R00207